SLING SUSPENSION THERAPY

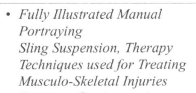

- *Fully Illustrated Manual Portraying Sling Suspension, Therapy Techniques used for Treating Musculo-Skeletal Injuries*
- *Extensive Section on Amputees*

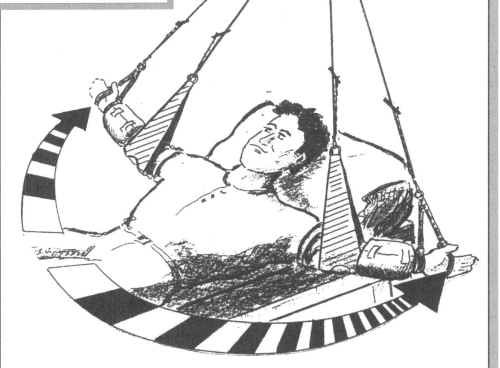

Text and Techniques by
John / George Barling, F.S.R.G.
Illustrations by Stan Wilkes

Order this book online at www.trafford.com
or email orders@trafford.com

Most Trafford titles are also available at major online book retailers.

Print information available on the last page.

ISBN: 978-1-5536-9581-3 (sc)
ISBN: 978-1-4122-4800-6 (e)

Trafford rev. 07/15/2019

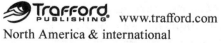 www.trafford.com
North America & international
toll-free: 1 888 232 4444 (USA & Canada)
fax: 812 355 4082

Contents

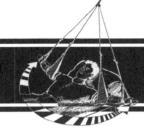

**Sling
Suspension
Therapy**

Foreword

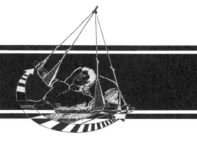

When joint motion is lost due to surgery or injury, a cure for restoring it presents a formidable challenge. No one method or combination of treatments can guarantee 100% return of motion beforehand. However, using Sling/cord suspension therapy techniques in association with other modalities provides the opportunity for obtaining some very good results. There is a great dearth of good, sound, practical information on this subject.

Having worked for some thirty-four years in rehabilitation centers in Canada and England where Sling/cord suspension is practiced, I have often wondered why the use of such techniques has invariably been passed on by word of mouth or by somebody else's lecture notes. At last Messrs. Barling and Wilkes have come to our aid. I highly recommend this manual to you for its clarity and the excellence of the illustrations. It attemps remarkably well to fill a void.

The author of the manual was first introduced to Sling Suspension in 1957 at Pinderfields General Hospital, Wakerfield, Yorkshire, England. As already noted, present literature on Sling/Cord Suspension is quite sparse and fragmented with but a cursory overview of the subject. It is important to note that the techniques illustrated in this manual have all been regularly used over a period of at least thirty years with gratifying success and significantly so in orthopaedic injuries and amputations. Several of the techniques are original and resulted from experimentation and the need to find safe and effective methods. The Cervical Series is original and the equipment required to perform three basic cervical movements is rudimentary but leaves room for improvement.

To the authors knowledge this is the first manual of its kind. It is certainly not the last word on the subject and it is hoped that others will aspire to improve on it with the passage of time. It is hoped that with the information illustrated, based on thirty years of continuous practice treating orthopaedic conditions will help to bridge the gap, and fill the present void on this subject.

Special thanks are extended to Mr. S. Wilkes for the long voluntary hours spent in illustrating this subject and to Mr. John George Barling for supplying the techniques and the text.

A.B. Kennard.

A.B. Kennard.M.B.,B.S. (Lond)

**Sling
Suspension
Therapy**

Preface

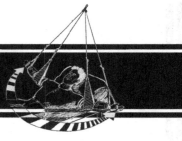

Sling suspension therapy is a well established form of physical therapy since it contributes towards the restoration of joint motion and tissue stretching. The principles explaining the subject of suspension therapy are described in several textbooks, but common to all is a lack of good illustrations accompanied by minimal text. The purpose is to illuminate and guide.

It would be presumptuous to think that this presentation has the answer to mobilizing all skeletal joints; neither does it profess to encompass the vast range, and sometimes subtle, sling and cord suspension techniques envisonable. The student and practitioner should find it helpful.

This paper is entirely original work and illustrates several new techniques not found in current literature.

Introduction

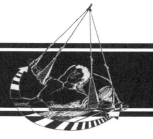

Selected techniques practiced daily and sometimes / accompanied by other physiotherapeutic treatment modalities have proven very beneficial for improving joint range as well as promoting stretch in soft tissues, especially in the treatment of Orthopaedic conditions.

Experience indicates that a 30 minute patient treatment session allows no more than two techniques to be beneficially applied if value for treatment is to be received. It also bears mentioning that one suspension technique employed for 25 minutes is well accepted by the patient, and at times more beneficial than several - particularly when treating acute and sub-acute conditions.

Moving the suspension point can result in a marked or subtle effect upon the motion. To increase joint range of motion (especially at the shoulder joint, but also applicable to several other joints), the important factor is sustained stretch at the limit of free motion up to the patient's tolerance.

Experience has shown that except in special circumstances swinging of the limb whilst in suspension has less effect upon gaining range of movement than a sustained stretch at the limit of free motion.

Correct placement of the overhead suspension point(s) is crucial for facilitating maximum pendular /oscillatory motion. It also determines whether the primary pendular motion receives assistance is relatively neutral or encounters resistance.

The capital letters A, N, R have been used in several illustrations to convey this principle.

A Represents the suspension point for ASSISTED pendular motion.

N Represents the suspension point for NEUTRAL pendular motion.

R Represents the suspension point for RESISTED pendular motion,

Nerve traction lesions to the upper and lower limbs can be treated with Sling Suspension. Gentle, slow controlled movement is taught to the patient and care not to over-stretch must be emphasized and observed. The Therapist will need to exercise patience and restraint.

Burns: Burn victims can derive good results from stretching in suspension when applied judiciously.

**Sling
Suspension
Therapy**

Equipment

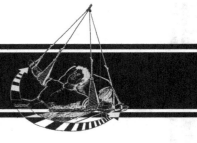

- Suspension Frame
- Various Slings
- Sling Dimensions
- Varied Supports

- Adjustable Weight and Pulley Frame Slide Clamp
- Shaped Heel Slings, Cords, Snaphooks and securing Strap
- Pulleys, Stopblock, Swivelhook and Sling Cord adjusters

Equipment necessary for effective Sling Suspension Therapy is listed under one of the four sub-groups mentioned below.

1. Suspension Cage / Frame

Suspension Cage and Frame should be devoid of sharp edges or corners. Metal burrs should be filed smooth. Two inch square meshing makes up the suspension caging welded at all points of corner contact, using TIG (Tungsten Inert Gas) method. A strong welded frame mesh results.

If a different sized Suspension Cage/Frame is contemplated, it is important that no space is lost or encroached upon, otherwise some suspension techniques might be stifled/crowded out.

Suspension frame side bars accomodate slidable metal clamps used for weight and pulley excercises. 5/8" diameter holes are drilled at 1-foot centers through the two side and one rear frame bar. These holes receive the metal pin that secures the clamp to the Horizontal Frames side/end bar(s) - The lowest edge of the frames mesh is positioned so it lies 8" (inches) above the top surface of the Frame Side and End Bars. (See illustrated Suspension Frame shown on Page 7).

2. Sling Cords - Slings - Attachments

A Sling suspension cord comprises a 1/4" diameter nylon cord with 2 sling swivel snap hooks and a wood slat threaded onto it. The wood slat has a hole at each end and facilitates easy shortening and lengthening of the cord. The spring catch of the snap hook(s) clip securely and safely to the roof mesh and permit of a common overhead suspension point from which 1,2,3 and even 4 suspension cords can arise. The use of the common overhead suspension point is exceedingly efficient accomodating smoothly to the changing planes of motion. A few techniques require several independant suspension points (see illustration). Caution: Do not suspend active equipment from S-hooks.

Sling Suspension Therapy

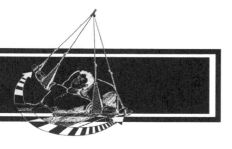

Sling design which needs to meet certain criteria before being adopted might include: sling shape, durability, flexibility, laundering effects, softness/texture, colored slings and slings with pockets that permit easy removal and replacement of sponge/rubber/silicone padding. The sling measurements given here have worked well for our needs.

Strap -like slings work very well for suspending feet and hands and result in a safe, snug suspension. Make certain the rings do not press into the soft tissue.

Some very tall or large men and women might require special slings. All suspension equipment can be hung on the side and rear mesh frames.

3. Sling Rings

Rings attached to slings should be strong. Functional use of the sling is improved if one ring can pass through another. The longer of the two strap-like slings provides a snug and safe suspension for the foot and ankle, the shorter for the hand and wrist but they are interchangeable, catering to large hands and small feet or vice-versa.

Large and small canvas heel slings provide a safe and secure alternative sling to the long, narrow, straplike slings and are simple to rig up.

Slings illustrated here are all used at one time or another. Measurements are provided for those wishing to make their own.
Note: The sling diagrams are not drawn to exact scale.

4. Dress/Clothing:

When using Suspension Therapy, the clothes worn should not interfere with motion. For the upper limb(s) and neck, a vest or t-shirt (with short sleeves) provides unrestricted range of movement. For lower limbs, shorts suffice. A track suit worn over the vest and shorts provides warmth and comfort. Clothing can be personal or provided by the rehabilitation center, sports medicine unit, or hospital etc. Clothing can be in the budget(s). A range of sizes, styles and colors should be available to accommodate tall, medium and short statured people.

Sling
Suspension
Therapy

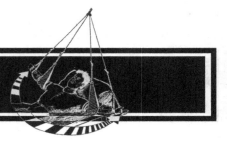

Footwear:

Runners are a good choice and in several suspension techniques they are left on the feet (foot); which permits a snugger fit in the sling - One can remove the runner but you have to be very adept at rigging the technique to avoid sock slippage that can result in a mal-aligned, uncomfortable sling.

Bandages:

Bandages are used to support, shape & shrink the stump.

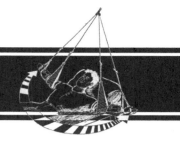

The Suspension Frame

2" Sqare Mesh TIG (Tungsten Inert Gas) welded at all contact corner points.

Standard wood plinth shown but hydraulic plinth preferred

**Sling, swivel, spring-snap hooks clip diagonally on to the corner(s) of the mesh.
This prevents the hook from sliding.**

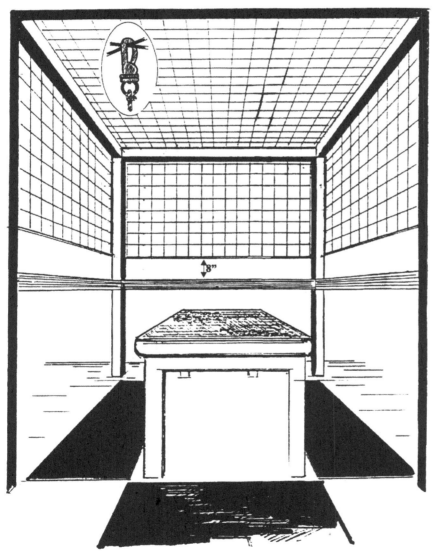

Frame Size

Height   7'

Depth   7'

Width   6'

Sling
Suspension
Therapy

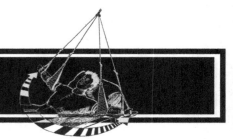

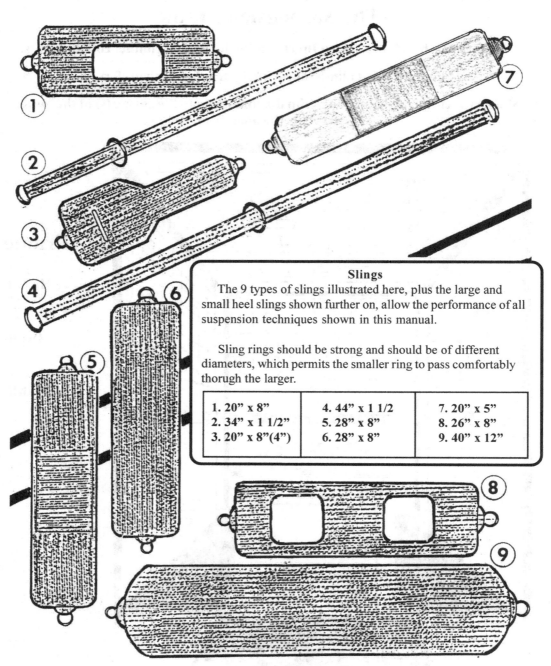

Slings

The 9 types of slings illustrated here, plus the large and small heel slings shown further on, allow the performance of all suspension techniques shown in this manual.

Sling rings should be strong and should be of different diameters, which permits the smaller ring to pass comfortably thorugh the larger.

1. 20" x 8"	4. 44" x 1 1/2	7. 20" x 5"
2. 34" x 1 1/2"	5. 28" x 8"	8. 26" x 8"
3. 20" x 8"(4")	6. 28" x 8"	9. 40" x 12"

Sling
Suspension
Therapy

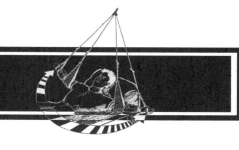

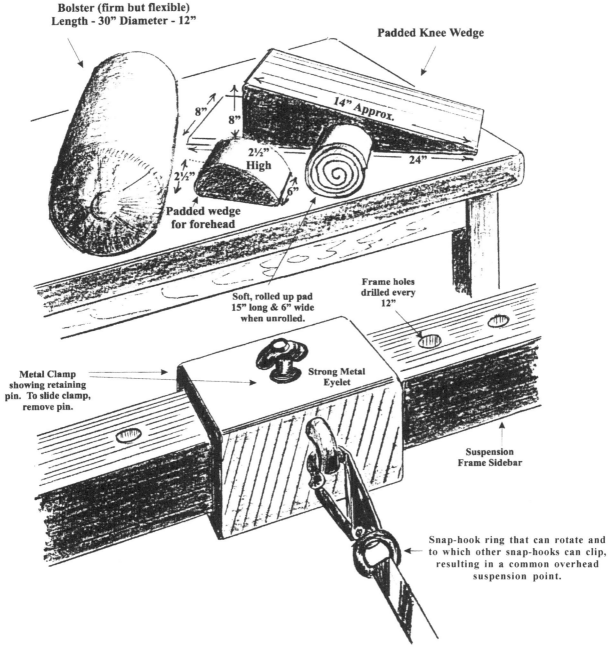

Bolster (firm but flexible)
Length - 30" Diameter - 12"

Padded Knee Wedge

8"

8"

14" Approx.

2½"
High

24"

2½"

6"

Padded wedge
for forehead

Frame holes
drilled every
12"

Soft, rolled up pad
15" long & 6" wide
when unrolled.

Metal Clamp
showing retaining
pin. To slide clamp,
remove pin.

Strong Metal
Eyelet

Suspension
Frame Sidebar

Snap-hook ring that can rotate and
to which other snap-hooks can clip,
resulting in a common overhead
suspension point.

Sling
Suspension
Therapy

9

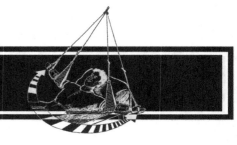

Note that a sling cord has two snap hooks. At one end, the cord is threaded through the eye of the swivel and securely tied. Thread the other cord end through one slat hole then through the eye of the snap hook and finally through the remaining slat hole. Tie a simple knot, the cord length is adjustable.

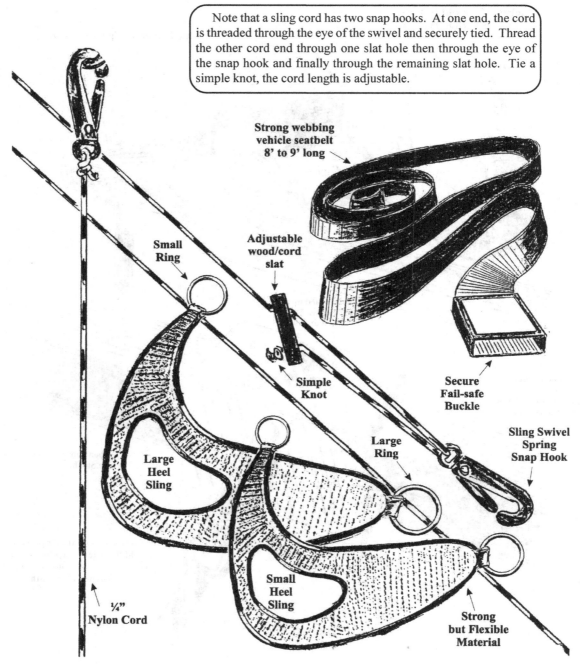

Strong webbing vehicle seatbelt 8' to 9' long

Small Ring

Adjustable wood/cord slat

Simple Knot

Secure Fail-safe Buckle

Sling Swivel Spring Snap Hook

Large Ring

Large Heel Sling

Small Heel Sling

¼" Nylon Cord

Strong but Flexible Material

Sling Suspension Therapy

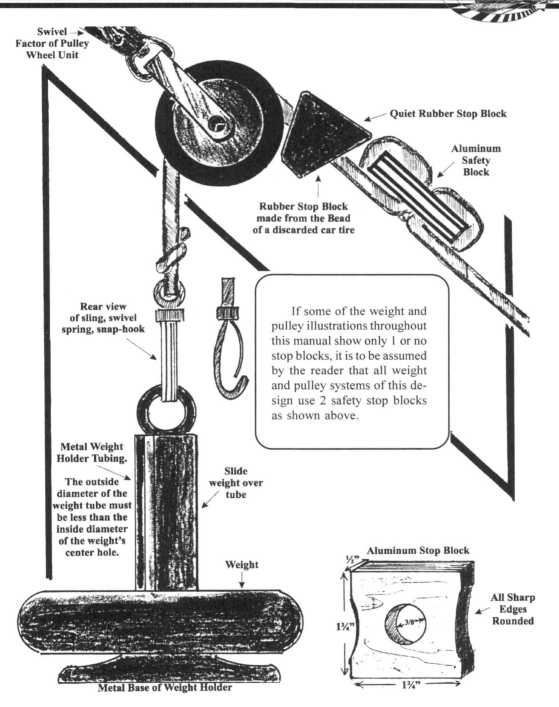

Swivel → Factor of Pulley Wheel Unit

Quiet Rubber Stop Block

Aluminum Safety Block

Rubber Stop Block made from the Bead of a discarded car tire

Rear view of sling, swivel spring, snap-hook

If some of the weight and pulley illustrations throughout this manual show only 1 or no stop blocks, it is to be assumed by the reader that all weight and pulley systems of this design use 2 safety stop blocks as shown above.

Metal Weight Holder Tubing.

The outside diameter of the weight tube must be less than the inside diameter of the weight's center hole.

Slide weight over tube

Weight

Metal Base of Weight Holder

Aluminum Stop Block

½"

1¾"

3/8"

1¾"

All Sharp Edges Rounded

Sling Suspension Therapy

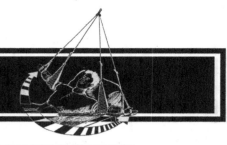

Snap Hooks

A. The Snap-hook clips over the crossed wires, which form the frames mesh. This safe/secure attachment prevents slippage of the clip along the frames wire.

B. Note the method used for adding or subtracting snap hooks/cord (see illustration below). This safe, snap hook, clipping system permits the use of up to 4 sling cords emanating out of (arising from) one common suspension point.

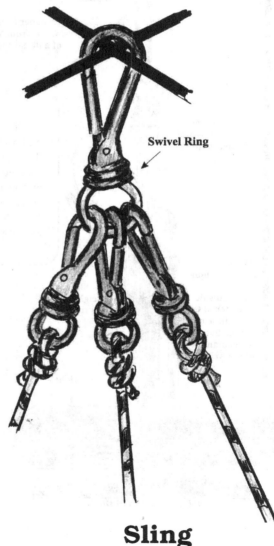

Swivel Ring

Sling Suspension Therapy

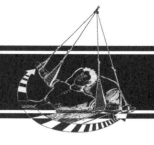

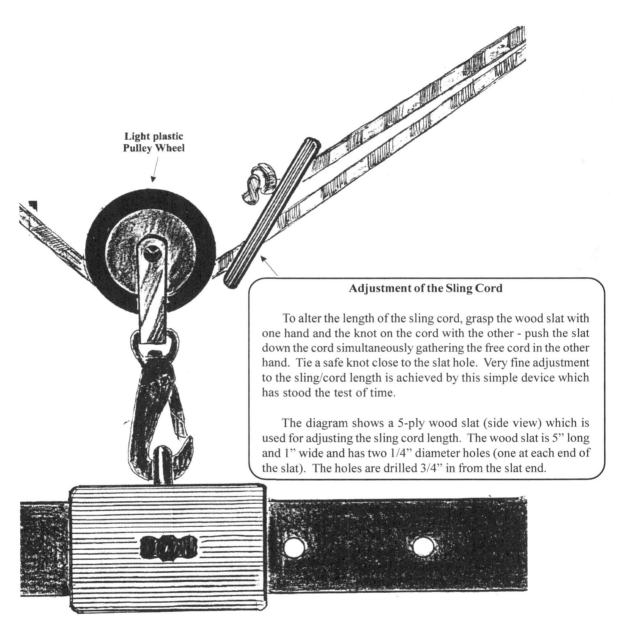

Light plastic Pulley Wheel

Adjustment of the Sling Cord

To alter the length of the sling cord, grasp the wood slat with one hand and the knot on the cord with the other - push the slat down the cord simultaneously gathering the free cord in the other hand. Tie a safe knot close to the slat hole. Very fine adjustment to the sling/cord length is achieved by this simple device which has stood the test of time.

The diagram shows a 5-ply wood slat (side view) which is used for adjusting the sling cord length. The wood slat is 5" long and 1" wide and has two 1/4" diameter holes (one at each end of the slat). The holes are drilled 3/4" in from the slat end.

Sling Suspension Therapy

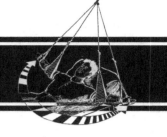

Illustrated Sling and Cord Suspension Therapy Techniques

Most Significant Factors

1. *Positioning of Patient*
2. *Appropriate Slings*
3. *Suitable supports*
4. *Methods of fixation*
5. *Range of motion control*
6. *Recommendations*
7. *Contra Indications*

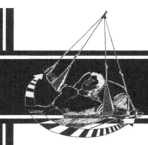
Cervical Series

Technique 1: Flexion / Extension

Technique 2: Rotation

Technique 3: Lateral Flexion

Technique 1:

CERVICAL FLEXION / EXTENSION

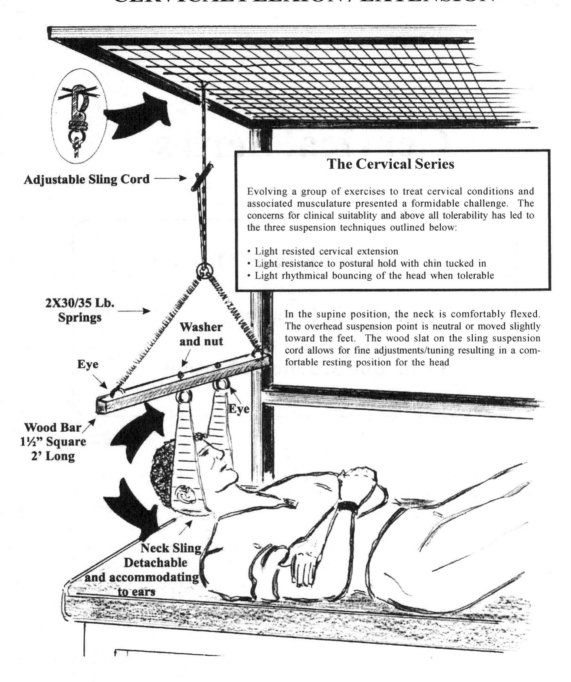

Adjustable Sling Cord →

2X30/35 Lb. Springs →

Washer and nut

Eye

Eye

Wood Bar 1½" Square 2' Long

Neck Sling Detachable and accommodating to ears

The Cervical Series

Evolving a group of exercises to treat cervical conditions and associated musculature presented a formidable challenge. The concerns for clinical suitablity and above all tolerability has led to the three suspension techniques outlined below:

• Light resisted cervical extension
• Light resistance to postural hold with chin tucked in
• Light rhythmical bouncing of the head when tolerable

In the supine position, the neck is comfortably flexed. The overhead suspension point is neutral or moved slightly toward the feet. The wood slat on the sling suspension cord allows for fine adjustments/tuning resulting in a comfortable resting position for the head

Sling Suspension Therapy

CERVICAL ROTATION / LATERAL FLEXIONS

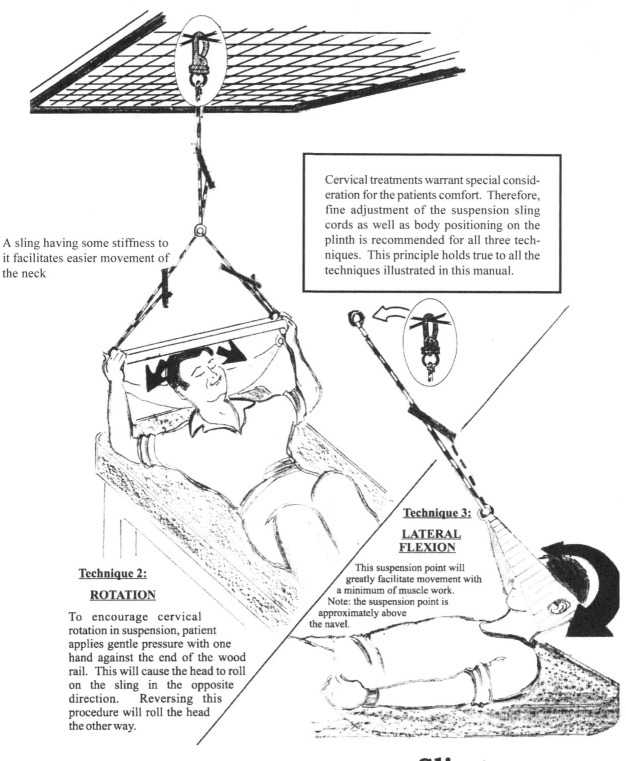

A sling having some stiffness to it facilitates easier movement of the neck

Cervical treatments warrant special consideration for the patients comfort. Therefore, fine adjustment of the suspension sling cords as well as body positioning on the plinth is recommended for all three techniques. This principle holds true to all the techniques illustrated in this manual.

Technique 3:

LATERAL FLEXION

This suspension point will greatly facilitate movement with a minimum of muscle work. Note: the suspension point is approximately above the navel.

Technique 2:

ROTATION

To encourage cervical rotation in suspension, patient applies gentle pressure with one hand against the end of the wood rail. This will cause the head to roll on the sling in the opposite direction. Reversing this procedure will roll the head the other way.

Sling Suspension Therapy

Arm & Shoulder-Girdle Series

Flexion & Extension (side lying)

(a) Abduction (bilateral) Assisted
(b) Abduction (bilateral) Neutral
(c) Abduction (bilateral) Resisted

Abduction (unilateral) Resisted

(a) Internal & External rotation (auto assist)
(b) External rotation (resisted)

Shoulder retraction (resisted)

Abduction/Adduction (bilateral)

Flexion through to Elevation

Arcs of movement (bilateral)
(a) Below shoulder level
(b) Approx. shoulder level
(c) Above shoulder level

Abduction (bilateral) Gravity and Weight assisted

Shoulder Flexion (bilateral) Auto Assisted Active Tension

**Sling
Suspension
Therapy**

SHOULDER FLEXION, SHOULDER EXTENSION (side lying)

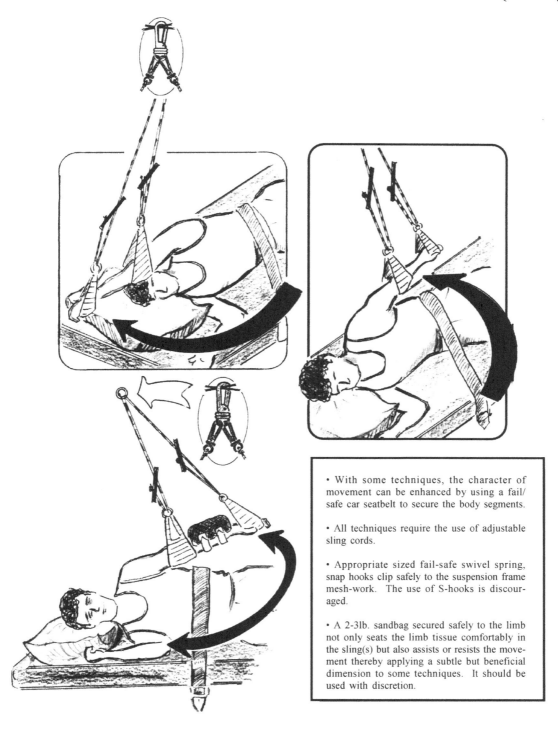

• With some techniques, the character of movement can be enhanced by using a fail/safe car seatbelt to secure the body segments.

• All techniques require the use of adjustable sling cords.

• Appropriate sized fail-safe swivel spring, snap hooks clip safely to the suspension frame mesh-work. The use of S-hooks is discouraged.

• A 2-3lb. sandbag secured safely to the limb not only seats the limb tissue comfortably in the sling(s) but also assists or resists the movement thereby applying a subtle but beneficial dimension to some techniques. It should be used with discretion.

**Sling
Suspension
Therapy**

SHOULDER ABDUCTION, (bilateral) ASSISTED

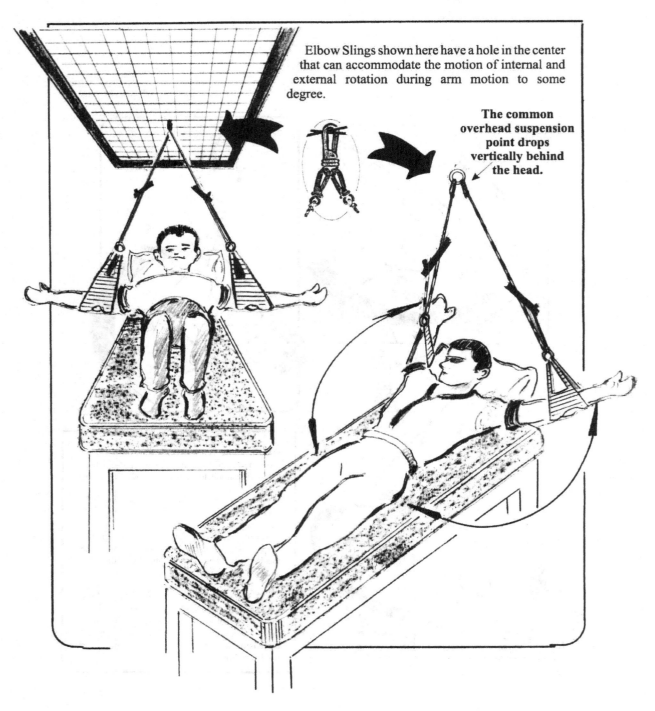

Elbow Slings shown here have a hole in the center that can accommodate the motion of internal and external rotation during arm motion to some degree.

The common overhead suspension point drops vertically behind the head.

**Sling
Suspension
Therapy**

20

SHOULDER ABDUCTION, (bilateral) NEUTRAL

Independent suspension from overhead.
Common suspension from overhead.

Moving the suspension point in front of or behind
the shoulder joint changes the demands on the
shoulder muscles from challenging to easy.

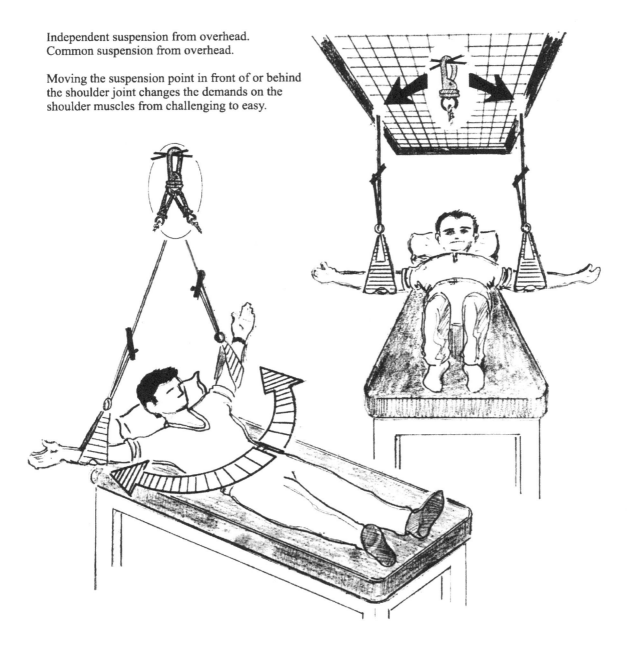

**Sling
Suspension
Therapy**

21

SHOULDER ABDUCTION, (Bilateral) RESISTED

- Swivel, spring clip, snap-hook of sling cord, shown clipped to sling ring.
- 2-3 lbs. sand bag held snugly to load forearm.
- Good use of a GM car seatbelt to stabilize the shoulder during resisted bi-lateral abduction of the arm.
- Common overhead suspension point located towards feet which will have resulted in very strong resistance to bilateral arm abduction.

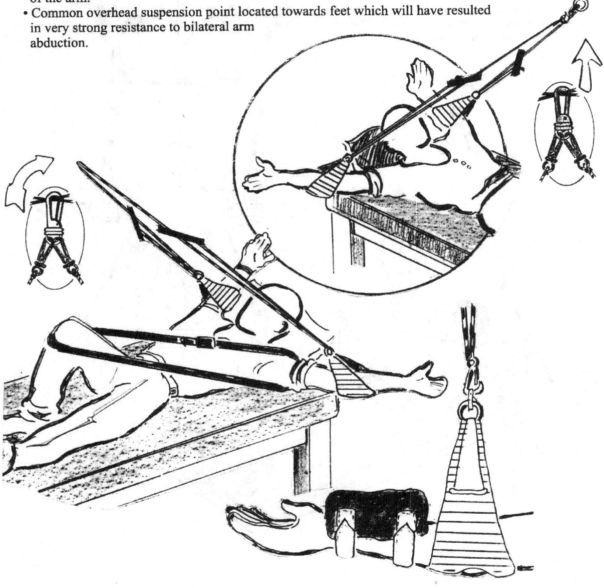

**Sling
Suspension
Therapy**

SHOULDER ABDUCTION, (Unilateral) RESISTED

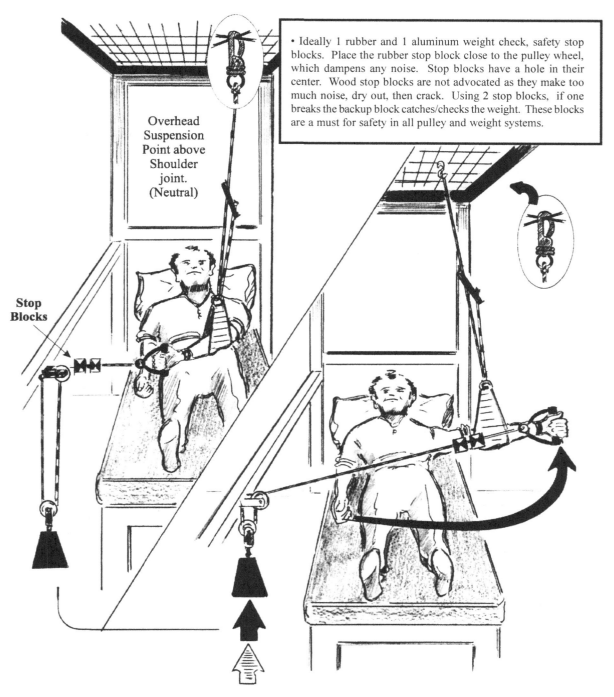

Overhead Suspension Point above Shoulder joint. (Neutral)

• Ideally 1 rubber and 1 aluminum weight check, safety stop blocks. Place the rubber stop block close to the pulley wheel, which dampens any noise. Stop blocks have a hole in their center. Wood stop blocks are not advocated as they make too much noise, dry out, then crack. Using 2 stop blocks, if one breaks the backup block catches/checks the weight. These blocks are a must for safety in all pulley and weight systems.

Stop Blocks

Sling Suspension Therapy

INTERNAL AND EXTERNAL ROTATIONS
AUTO & WEIGHT ASSISTED

Upper arm supported at 90° abduction. Active internal and external upper arm rotation utilizing active, eccentric and concentric muscle work. The weight of the hand and forearm might be said to act as weight resistance that alters and is greatest when the forearm is horizontal to the ground. For most of the range, the sandbag added to the forearm, wants to push it to internal rotation.

Note: The independant suspension cord and sling illustrated below, 1 lb progressing to 5lbs. is sufficient sandbag weight.

The upper arm should have 90° abduction to use the techniques shown here.

The overhead suspension is above the center of the upper arm (neutral)

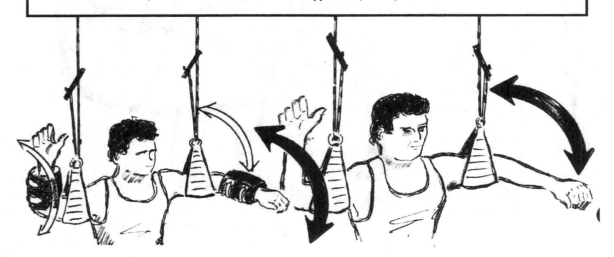

**Sling
Suspension
Therapy**

INTERNAL AND EXTERNAL ROTATIONS
AUTO & WEIGHT ASSISTED

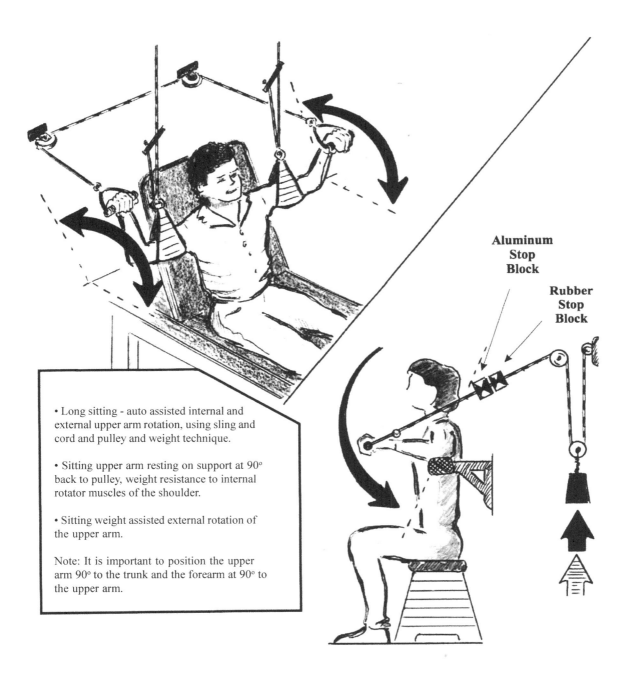

Aluminum
Stop
Block

Rubber
Stop
Block

• Long sitting - auto assisted internal and external upper arm rotation, using sling and cord and pulley and weight technique.

• Sitting upper arm resting on support at 90° back to pulley, weight resistance to internal rotator muscles of the shoulder.

• Sitting weight assisted external rotation of the upper arm.

Note: It is important to position the upper arm 90° to the trunk and the forearm at 90° to the upper arm.

**Sling
Suspension
Therapy**

SHOULDER RETRACTION (Unilateral Resisted)

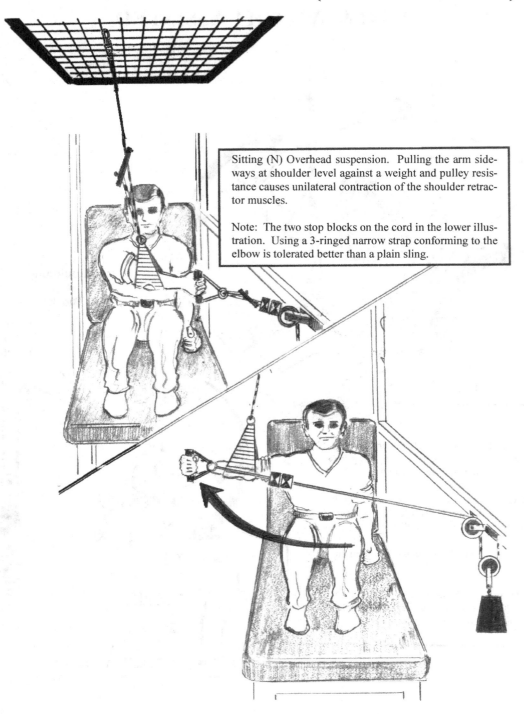

Sitting (N) Overhead suspension. Pulling the arm sideways at shoulder level against a weight and pulley resistance causes unilateral contraction of the shoulder retractor muscles.

Note: The two stop blocks on the cord in the lower illustration. Using a 3-ringed narrow strap conforming to the elbow is tolerated better than a plain sling.

Sling
Suspension
Therapy

SHOULDER ABDUCTION/ ADDUCTION (Bilateral)

The illustrations depict several positions whilst lying prone. A supportive wedge has proven beneficial for comfort and occasionally facilitates the exercise. The subsidiary motion of lumbar extension/hyper-extension enhances the pattern of movement. The handles suspended from the sling cords should just graze the top of the plinth when first introducing the exercise. Attention should be directed to the lumbar spine when necessary, many patients are comfortable without lumbar supports. All techniques shown use a common overhead suspension point and sling cords.

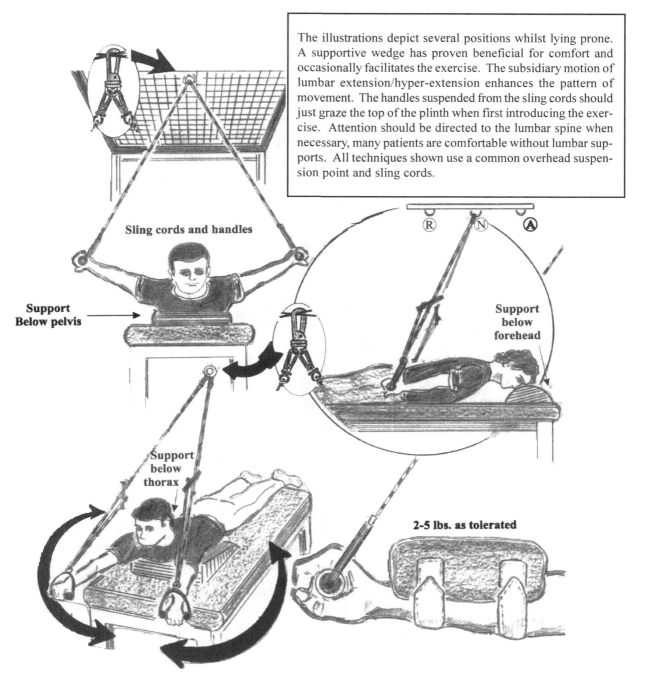

Sling cords and handles

Support Below pelvis

Ⓡ Ⓝ Ⓐ

Support below forehead

Support below thorax

2-5 lbs. as tolerated

Sling Suspension Therapy

SHOULDER FLEXION THROUGH TO ELEVATION

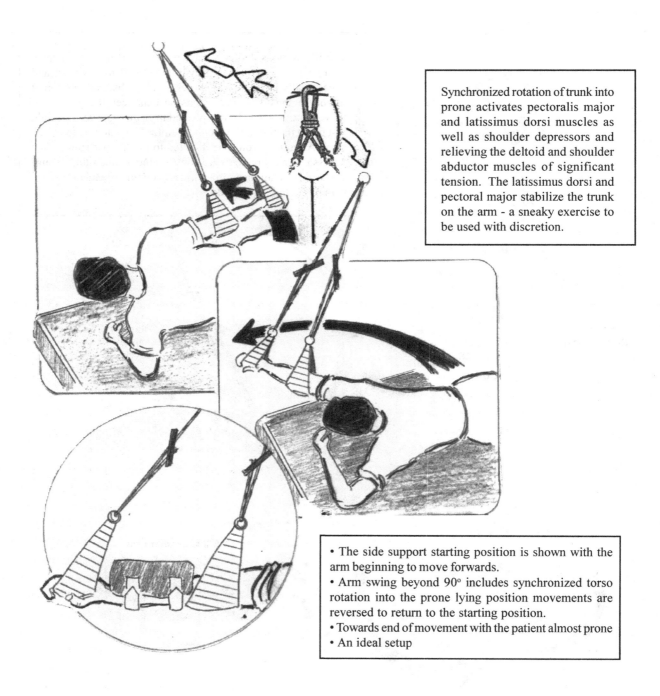

Synchronized rotation of trunk into prone activates pectoralis major and latissimus dorsi muscles as well as shoulder depressors and relieving the deltoid and shoulder abductor muscles of significant tension. The latissimus dorsi and pectoral major stabilize the trunk on the arm - a sneaky exercise to be used with discretion.

• The side support starting position is shown with the arm beginning to move forwards.
• Arm swing beyond 90° includes synchronized torso rotation into the prone lying position movements are reversed to return to the starting position.
• Towards end of movement with the patient almost prone
• An ideal setup

ARCS OF SHOULDER MOVEMENT
Below Shoulder Level (Bilateral)

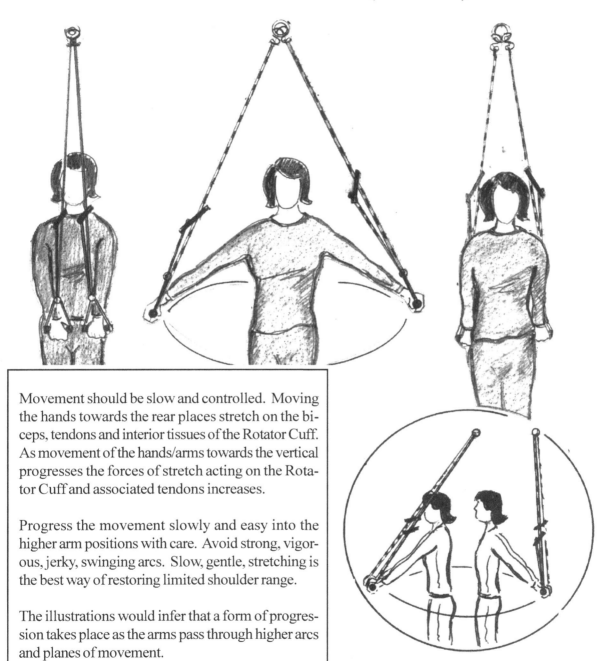

Movement should be slow and controlled. Moving the hands towards the rear places stretch on the biceps, tendons and interior tissues of the Rotator Cuff. As movement of the hands/arms towards the vertical progresses the forces of stretch acting on the Rotator Cuff and associated tendons increases.

Progress the movement slowly and easy into the higher arm positions with care. Avoid strong, vigorous, jerky, swinging arcs. Slow, gentle, stretching is the best way of restoring limited shoulder range.

The illustrations would infer that a form of progression takes place as the arms pass through higher arcs and planes of movement.

ARCS OF SHOULDER MOVEMENT
At Shoulder Level (Bilateral)

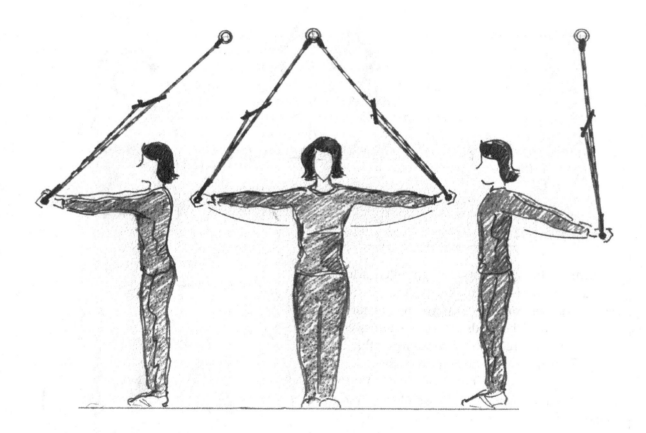

Note the wood slats on the sling cords for raising or lowering the arms/handles. A pulley or common overhead, fixed point may be used to perform this technique. A fixed common, overhead point is preferred.

Sling
Suspension
Therapy

ARCS OF SHOULDER MOVEMENT
Above Shoulder Level (Bilateral)

Notice in the illustration below that the patient, by stepping ahead of the overhead, fixed, common point causes the arms to lift well above the shoulder level in
a high low arching movement.

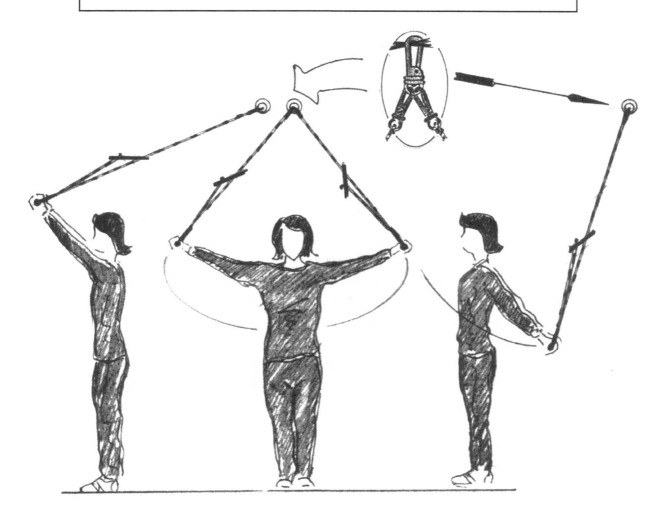

Sling
Suspension
Therapy

ABDUCTION (Bilateral) GRAVITY & WEIGHT ASSISTED

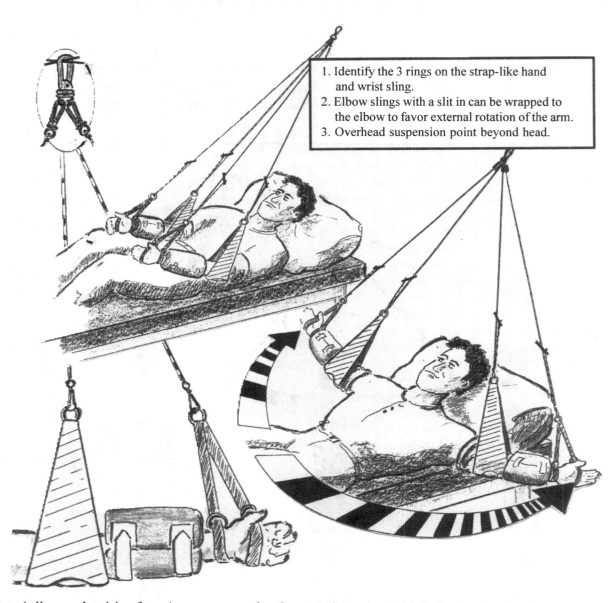

1. Identify the 3 rings on the strap-like hand and wrist sling.
2. Elbow slings with a slit in can be wrapped to the elbow to favor external rotation of the arm.
3. Overhead suspension point beyond head.

Note 4 sling cords arising from 1 common overhead suspension point. Initially both arms might be suspended 45° to 50° of shoulder flexion. To obtain abduction, allow both arms to move out sidewards and upwards. Shoulder retractor muscles may assist the abductors in this motion. The pectorals might work eccentrically to dampen the speed of motion. To gain pure bilateral shoulder abduction, suspend both arms in less flexion until the slings come to lie alongside the body. Moving the arms sideways in this position will result in true bilateral arm and shoulder abduction.

**Sling
Suspension
Therapy**

SHOULDER FLEXION (Bilateral)
AUTOASSISTED ACTIVE TENSION

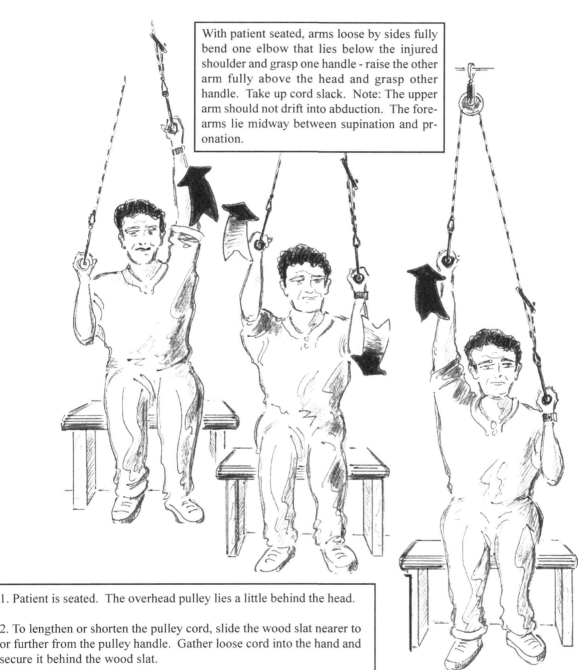

With patient seated, arms loose by sides fully bend one elbow that lies below the injured shoulder and grasp one handle - raise the other arm fully above the head and grasp other handle. Take up cord slack. Note: The upper arm should not drift into abduction. The forearms lie midway between supination and pronation.

1. Patient is seated. The overhead pulley lies a little behind the head.

2. To lengthen or shorten the pulley cord, slide the wood slat nearer to or further from the pulley handle. Gather loose cord into the hand and secure it behind the wood slat.

Note: Correct positioning of the patient and precise pulley cord adjustment is imperative. See hand and arm position illustrated in the 1st & 3rd diagrams above.

Sling Suspension Therapy

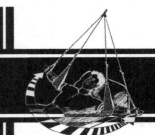

Part ③

Lumbar Spine Series

Bilateral Lateral Trunk Flexions in Supine Suspension

Shoulder and Upper Trunk Partially Fixed

Bilateral Lateral Trunk Flexions in Supine Suspension

Leg and Pelvis partially fixed

**Sling
Suspension
Therapy**

BILATERAL LATERAL TRUNK FLEXIONS
IN SUPINE SUSPENSION
SHOULDER & UPPER TRUNK PARTIALLY FIXED

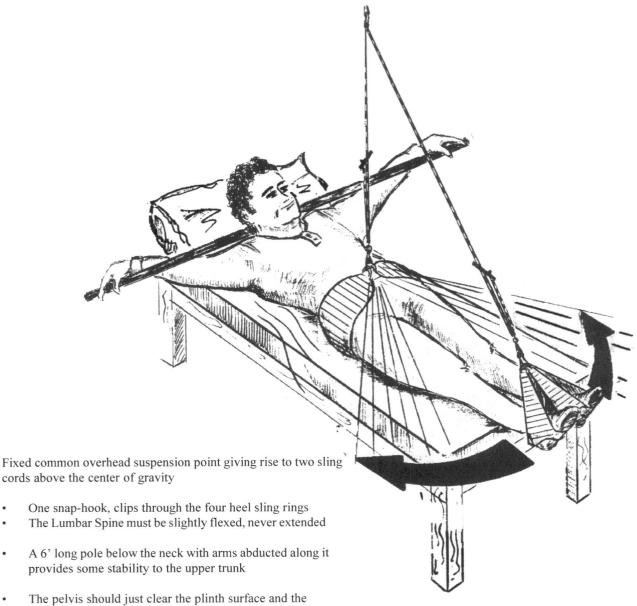

Fixed common overhead suspension point giving rise to two sling cords above the center of gravity

- One snap-hook, clips through the four heel sling rings
- The Lumbar Spine must be slightly flexed, never extended

- A 6' long pole below the neck with arms abducted along it provides some stability to the upper trunk

- The pelvis should just clear the plinth surface and the Lumbar Spine neutral or slightly flexed

- Activate the hip and trunk side flexors gradually increasing the Arc of Motion

- If the legs and pelvis rotate recheck your rigging

**Sling
Suspension
Therapy**

BILATERAL LATERAL TRUNK FLEXIONS
IN SUPINE SUSPENSION
(Includes fixation of abducted legs)

Fixed common overhead suspension point giving rise to three sling cords above the center of gravity

- Feet are securely tied to side frame.

- The Lumbar Spine must be slightly flexed, never extended

- The relative fixation of the legs on the pelvis provide a base for performing Bilateral trunk side flexion

- The legs must remain straight during the exercise. A side benefit to this exercise is the strong action played by the hip abductor muscles towards fixation of the pelvis.

- The knees remain straight during the exercise.

- If trunk rotates recheck your rigging

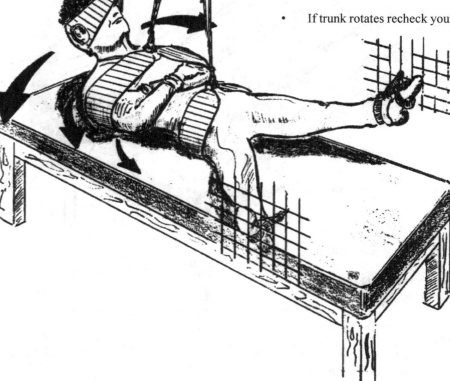

Sling
Suspension
Therapy

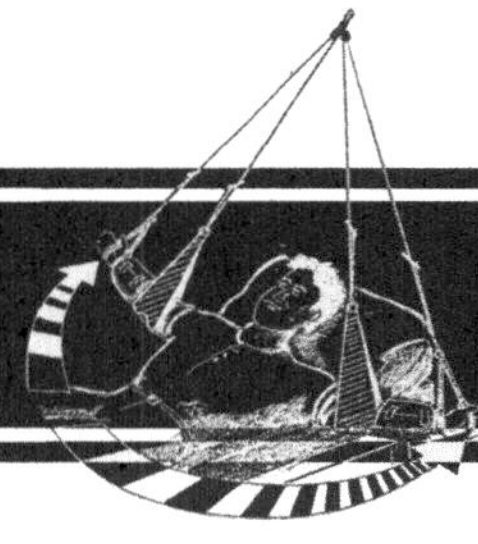

Part 4

Hip Joint Series

<u>**ABDUCTION**</u>

Free Movement (unilateral)

Free Movement (bilateral)

Resisted Movement (unilateral)

Resisted Movement (bilateral)

<u>**EXTENSION**</u>

Free Movement (unilateral side lying)

Resisted Movement (unilateral side lying)

Resisted Movement (unilateral supine)

Resisted Movement Unilateral (supine)

Resisted Movement (bilateral supine)

Adductor & Hamstring stretching (bilateral) Long Sitting

Bi-Lateral Hip, Knee Flexion Long Sitting

**Sling
Suspension
Therapy**

UNILATERAL FREE MOVEMENT

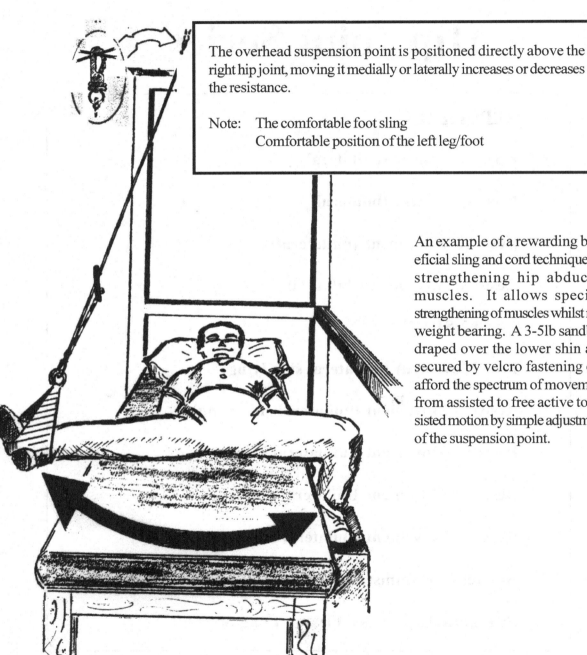

The overhead suspension point is positioned directly above the right hip joint, moving it medially or laterally increases or decreases the resistance.

Note: The comfortable foot sling
        Comfortable position of the left leg/foot

An example of a rewarding beneficial sling and cord technique for strengthening hip abductor muscles. It allows specific strengthening of muscles whilst non weight bearing. A 3-5lb sandbag draped over the lower shin and secured by velcro fastening can afford the spectrum of movement from assisted to free active to resisted motion by simple adjustment of the suspension point.

Sling
Suspension
Therapy

BILATERAL FREE MOVEMENT

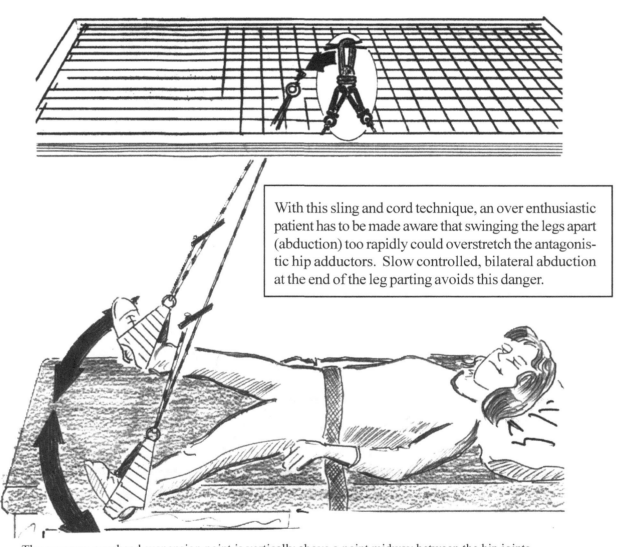

With this sling and cord technique, an over enthusiastic patient has to be made aware that swinging the legs apart (abduction) too rapidly could overstretch the antagonistic hip adductors. Slow controlled, bilateral abduction at the end of the leg parting avoids this danger.

The common overhead suspension point is vertically above a point midway between the hip joints.

Moving the overhead point towards the foot or head increases or decreases the resistance.

Note: Strapping a 2-5lb. sandbag to the ankle(s) helps to seat the foot snugly in the sling and provides a form of resistance.

UNILATERAL RESISTED MOVEMENT

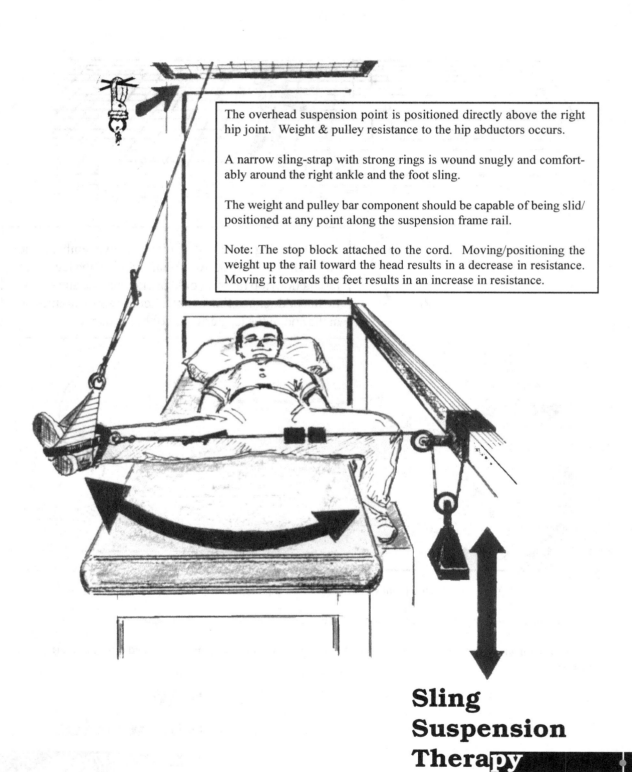

The overhead suspension point is positioned directly above the right hip joint. Weight & pulley resistance to the hip abductors occurs.

A narrow sling-strap with strong rings is wound snugly and comfortably around the right ankle and the foot sling.

The weight and pulley bar component should be capable of being slid/positioned at any point along the suspension frame rail.

Note: The stop block attached to the cord. Moving/positioning the weight up the rail toward the head results in a decrease in resistance. Moving it towards the feet results in an increase in resistance.

**Sling
Suspension
Therapy**

BILATERAL RESISTED MOVEMENT

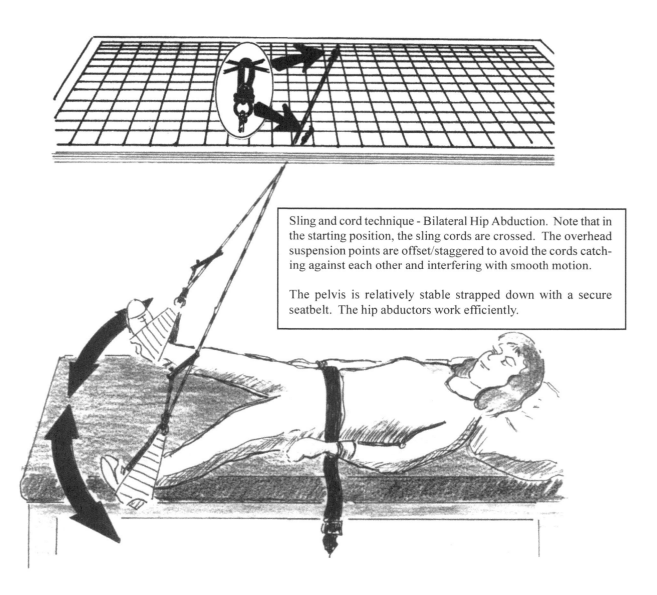

Sling and cord technique - Bilateral Hip Abduction. Note that in the starting position, the sling cords are crossed. The overhead suspension points are offset/staggered to avoid the cords catching against each other and interfering with smooth motion.

The pelvis is relatively stable strapped down with a secure seatbelt. The hip abductors work efficiently.

Positioning the offset, overhead suspension points above the ankles produces a good action for bilateral hip abductor muscle strengthening - securing a 2-5 lb sandbag around each ankle produces and permits a gradual increase in resistance to the movement.

Sling
Suspension
Therapy

UNILATERAL SIDE LYING FREE MOVEMENT

The overhead suspension point is positioned vertically above the hip joint, moving the suspension point in front of or behind the hip resists or assists hip extension.

The emphasis is on hip hypertension. The leg motion should be slow, steady and controlled.

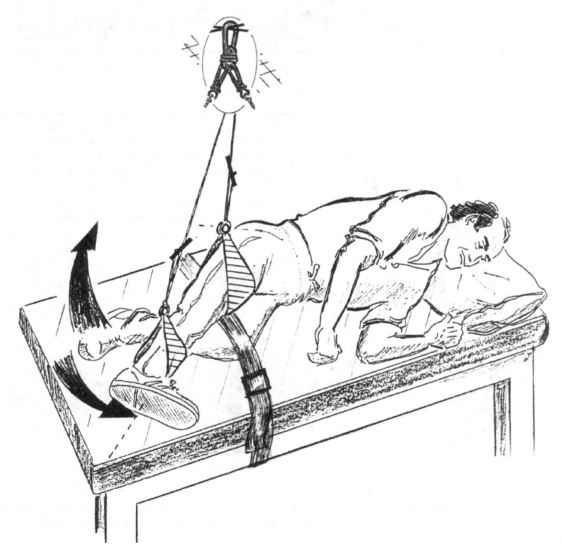

UNILATERAL SIDE LYING WEIGHT RESISTANCE

A common overhead suspension point of the two sling cords. Attempt to hyper-extend the hip.

A narrow sling-strap with strong rings (not illustrated) can support the foot comfortably and snugly, sometimes preferable to a plain sling. Motion should be smooth and controlled.

The weight can be slid into any position along the suspension frame bar, and subtly affects the resistance which lessens as you slide it towards the head.

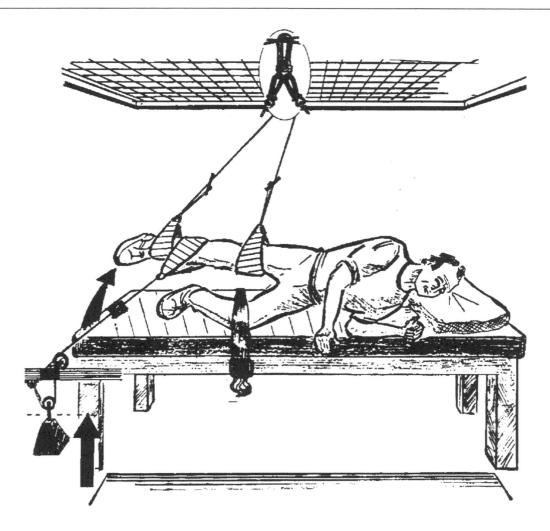

**Sling
Suspension
Therapy**

UNILATERAL SUPINE LYING WEIGHT RESISTANCE

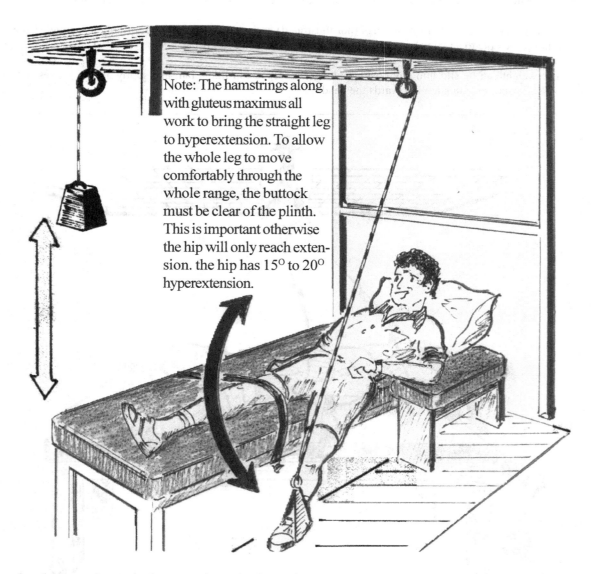

Note: The hamstrings along with gluteus maximus all work to bring the straight leg to hyperextension. To allow the whole leg to move comfortably through the whole range, the buttock must be clear of the plinth. This is important otherwise the hip will only reach extension. the hip has 15° to 20° hyperextension.

The overhead suspension point is approximately above the head moving it towards the feet subtly increases the resistance.

Note: The restraining strap on the right knee.

**Sling
Suspension
Therapy**

UNILATERAL SUPINE WEIGHT RESISTANCE

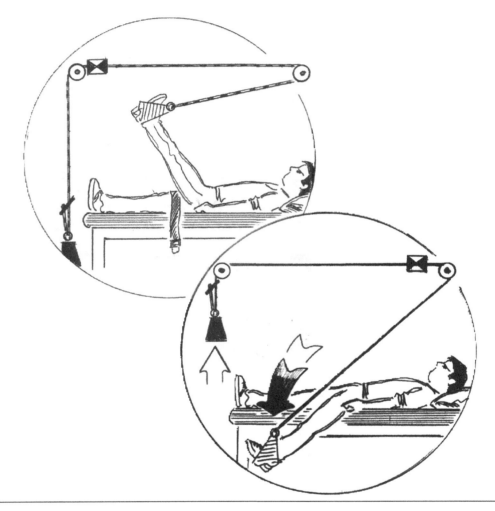

Note: The stop blocks to check the weight.

Excellent illustration of weight resistance during hip hyperextension in the frontal plane from nearly full outer to full inner range.

Not all weight and pulley illustrations show the two stop blocks for catching the weight, but it should be assumed this safety feature will be applied in practice.

**Sling
Suspension
Therapy**

BILATERAL SUPINE WEIGHT RESISTANCE

The overhead suspension point is not critical, but usually positioned between the hips and the head-the two foot slings slip on to the weight cord. A strap holds the hips down.

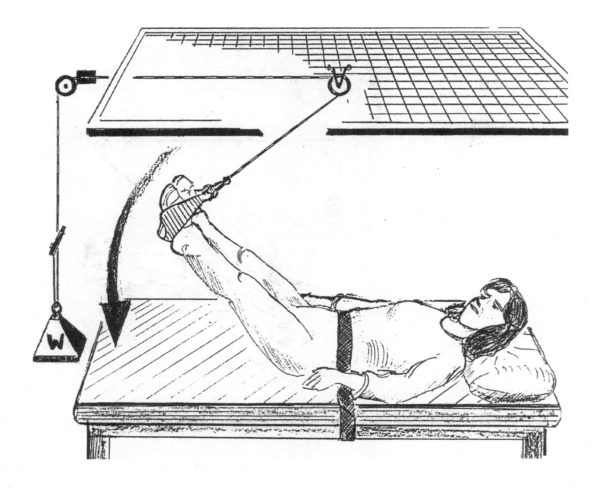

**Sling
Suspension
Therapy**

BILATERAL HIP ADDUCTOR AND HAMSTRING TENDON STRETCHING

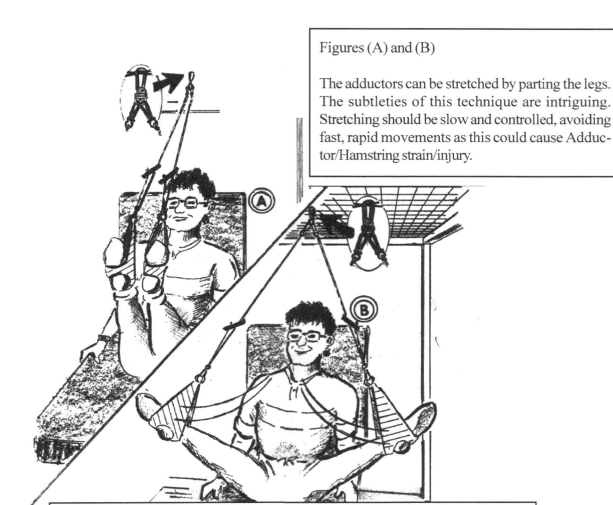

Figures (A) and (B)

The adductors can be stretched by parting the legs. The subtleties of this technique are intriguing. Stretching should be slow and controlled, avoiding fast, rapid movements as this could cause Adductor/Hamstring strain/injury.

Adjust the back support on a plinth to permit comfortable long sitting. Suspend the legs in two heel slings. The common overhead suspension point is situated a little behind the head. Figure (A) shows hamstring stretching and figure (B) Adductor muscle stretching. To increase the stretch, bend both knees, figure (C), and move the wood slats up the cord towards the overhead suspension point.

Sling Suspension Therapy

BILATERAL HIP AND KNEE FLEXION

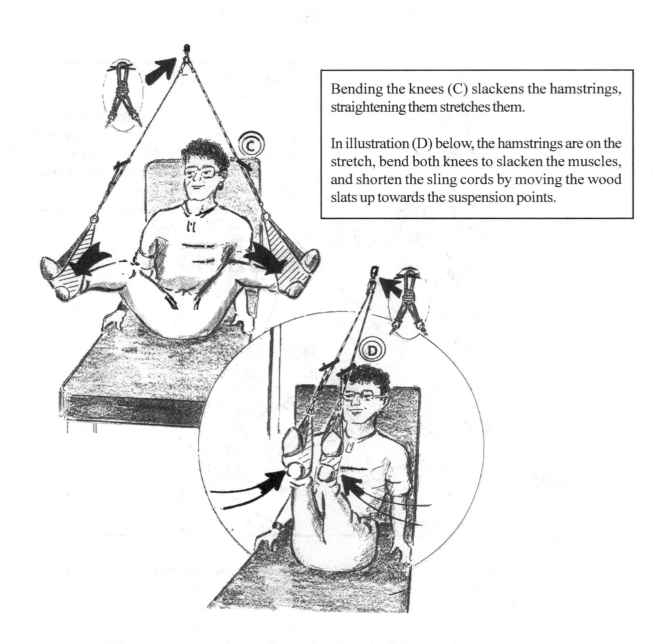

Bending the knees (C) slackens the hamstrings, straightening them stretches them.

In illustration (D) below, the hamstrings are on the stretch, bend both knees to slacken the muscles, and shorten the sling cords by moving the wood slats up towards the suspension points.

**Sling
Suspension
Therapy**

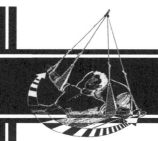

Knee Joint Series

PART A - Extensions

K1   (A) **Starting Position**
        (B) **Knee Extension**
        (C) **Knee Extension with S.L.R.**

K2   (A) **Long Sitting weight assisted**
        (B) **Knee Extension - As arm raises weight**
            transfers to knee

K3   (A) **Weight Assisted Knee - Extension Prone Lying**
        (B) **Weight Assists knee extension as pulley handle rises**

K4   (A) **Prone Lying - Active, concentric quads muscle**
            strengthening. Weight pulley resistance.
        (B) **Prone Lying - A weight pulley excercise to strengthen**
            the quadriceps.

Sling
Suspension
Therapy

WEIGHT RESISTANCE LONG SITTING

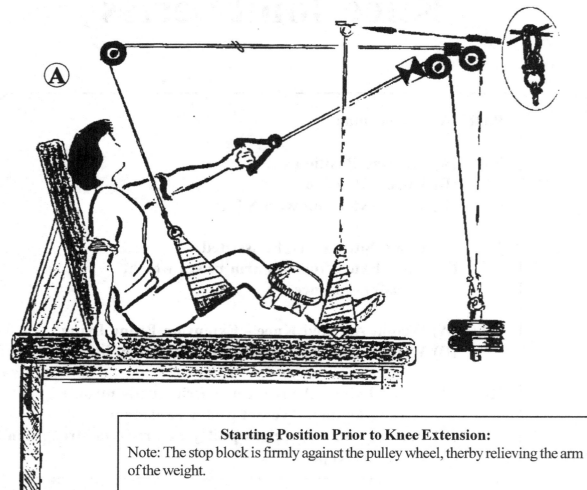

Starting Position Prior to Knee Extension:

Note: The stop block is firmly against the pulley wheel, therby relieving the arm of the weight.

Illustrations (A), (B) and (C) make demands upon hip, thigh and dorsiflexor muscles of the foot. The sandbag (2-5lbs) not only helps to seat the heel in the sling, but acts as a resistance to the thigh muscle during straight leg lifting. The illustration speaks for itself.

**Sling
Suspension
Therapy**

LONG SITTING UNILATERAL WEIGHT RESISTANCE

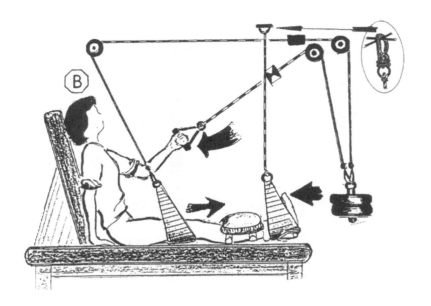

Utilizing the hip extensor and hamstring muscles, the knee extends (straightens). The pulley arm now holds the weight and bends to take up the slack in the cord- the foot is dorsi-flexed. Arrows indicate the direction of movement.

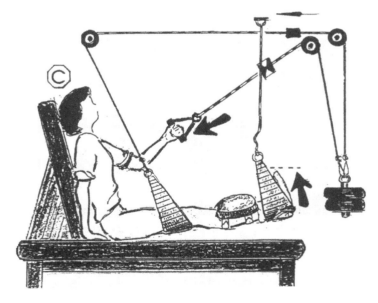

Active knee extension occurs by contraction of the quadricep(s) muscle, simultaneously dorsi-flexing the foot and lifting the straight leg. Note: The pulley arm is now holding all the weight. To return to the starting position, straighten the pulley arm easing the weight on to the stop block and bend the hip and knee.

Sling Suspension Therapy

WEIGHT ASSISTED (SITTING)

In this illustration, the knee is slightly flexed and the weight is held/controlled by the hand. The next illustration shows the arm raising/transferring the weight on to the knee.

Note: Two slings are used for this technique.

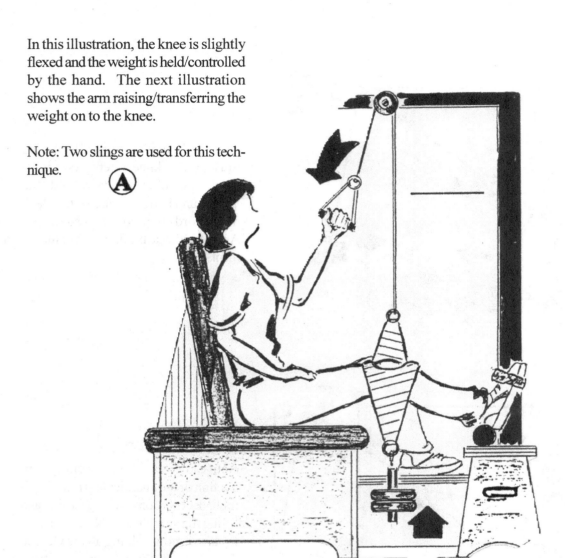

A useful technique for stretching the medial and lateral ligs of the knee following injury after all other efforts to extend it have been exhausted. Positioning of the patient must be correct and the slings positioned accurately. A knee extension lag can often be rectified by strengthening of the quads muscle but if this fails due to damaged ligs with possible thickening and binding of these structures, the technique shown here is sometimes successful when performed in conjunction with the technique illustrated on Pages 54 and 56. The hole in the sling must permit free motion of the Patella. Be very careful removing and adding weights. Increase weight by 2-1/2 lbs. increments to tolerable level(s).

WEIGHT ASSISTED (SITTING)

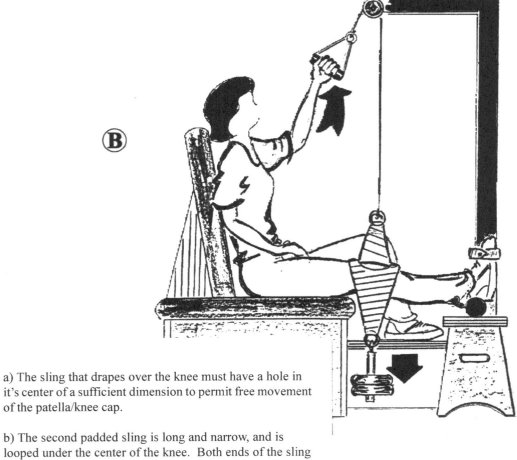

Ⓑ

a) The sling that drapes over the knee must have a hole in it's center of a sufficient dimension to permit free movement of the patella/knee cap.

b) The second padded sling is long and narrow, and is looped under the center of the knee. Both ends of the sling emerge through the other sling as illustrated. It is imperative that this technique uses the correct fitting slings. Comfort is of paramount importance.

c) The foot is strapped in the neutral position to the suspension frame with the heel resting on a pad/stool.

d) Experience has shown that 10-30lb is tolerated for short periods of time depending on body type and pain tolerance factors. Caution must be observed when attaching and detaching the weighted bar to the sling rings.

e) The hip and knee extend whilst the forefoot actively dorsi-flexes as weight is transferred from the hand to the knee.

WEIGHT ASSISTED (PRONE LYING)

The illustration shows the arm/hand holding the weight and the knee relaxed. The foot strapped securely to the suspension frame and the hips held down securely.

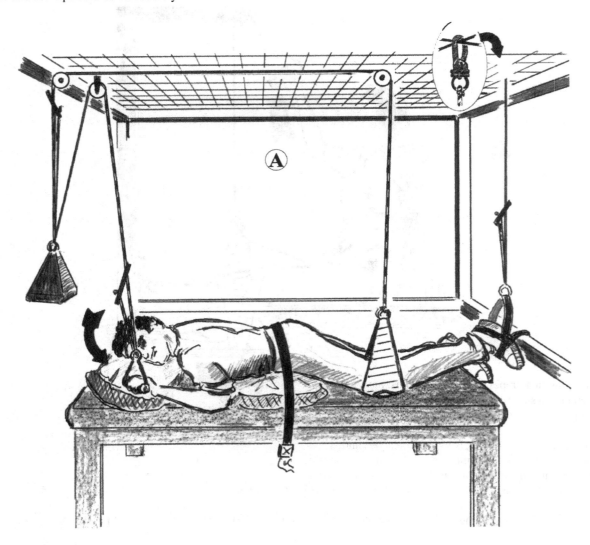

A useful alternative technique for stretching knee flexion contractures

WEIGHT ASSISTED (PRONE LYING)

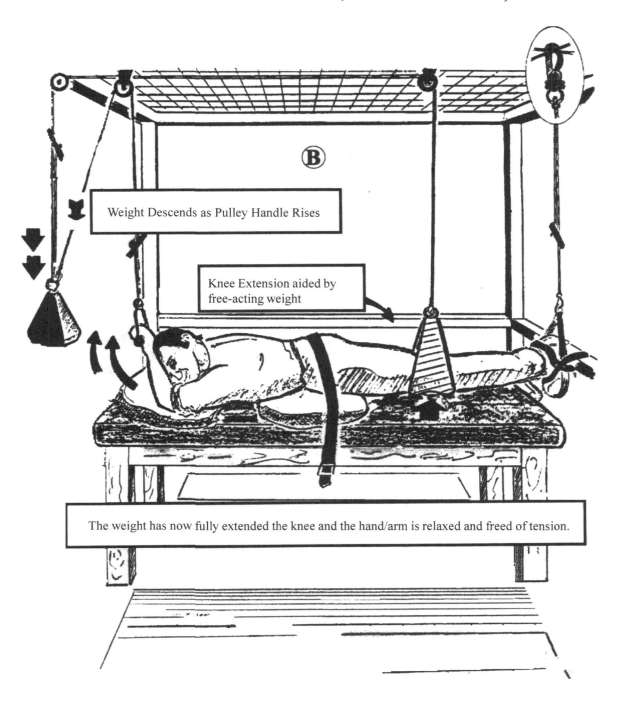

B

Weight Descends as Pulley Handle Rises

Knee Extension aided by free-acting weight

The weight has now fully extended the knee and the hand/arm is relaxed and freed of tension.

Sling Suspension Therapy

WEIGHT RESISTED (PRONE LYING)

A foot sling is shown in the illustrations. A strong, narrow strap sling can also be used which permits a snug and comfortable wrap to the ankle. Notice the sling support holding the thigh and the belt securing the hips. Straightening of the leg results in a strong contraction of the quadriceps muscle including the rectus femoris. Hip flexors to some degree work as fixator muscles. The stop block as it engages the pulley, carries the weight thereby permitting the leg to relax.

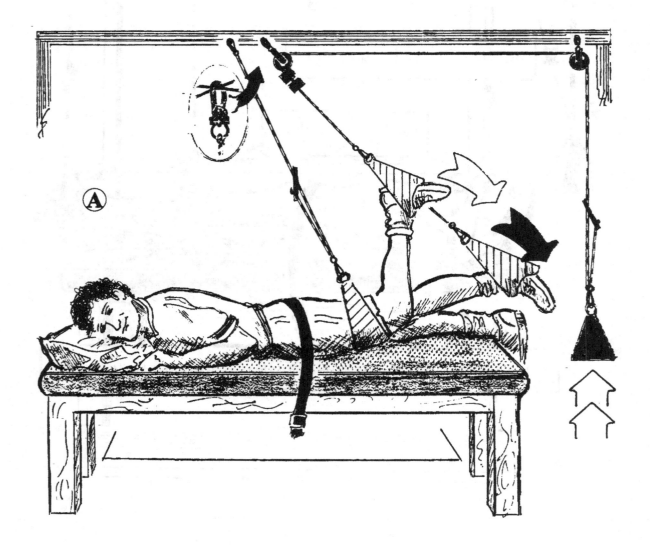

**Sling
Suspension
Therapy**

WEIGHT RESISTED (PRONE LYING)

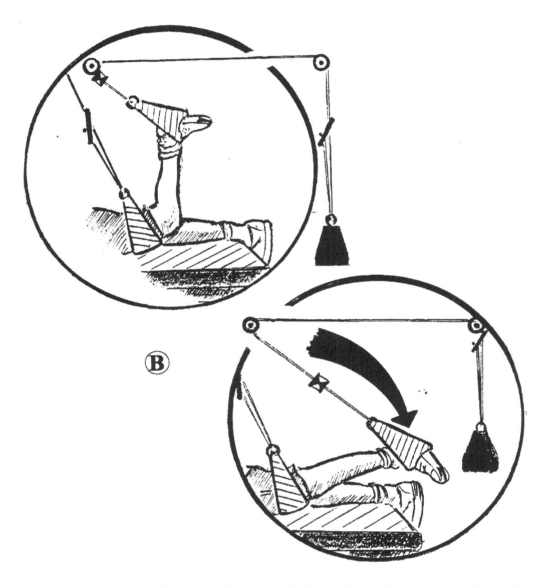

B

In the starting position, the thigh is held hyperextended by a sling cord. A separate pulley and weight and ankle sling allow the knee to be held well-flexed (see adjacent page). Placing all the thigh muscles on the stretch including Rectus Femoris prepares the muscles, physiologically, for strong contraction.

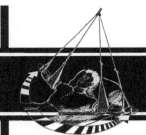

Knee Joint Series

PART B - Flexions

Sling Suspension Therapy

WEIGHT & GRAVITY ASSISTED
(SUPINE LYING)

The overhead suspension point should be such that it permits the knee to fully bend without obstruction from the pulley cord. Illustration A shows the overhead suspension point above the head that is acceptable in the majority of cases.

Illustration B and C illustrate the movement.

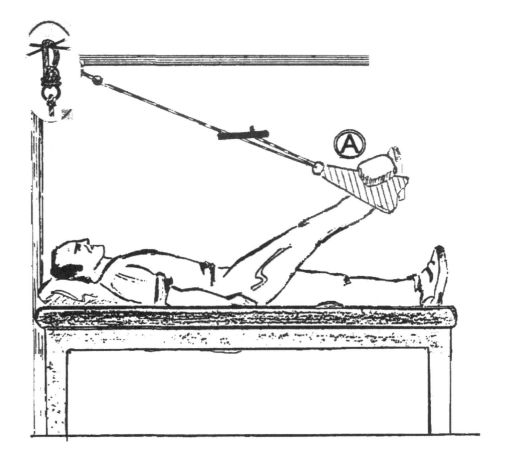

The sandbag draped over the foot sling helps to snug the heel into the sling and working with gravity results in a weight-assisted knee flexion and weight-resisted knee extension.

Sling
Suspension
Therapy

WEIGHT & GRAVITY ASSISTED
(SUPINE LYING)

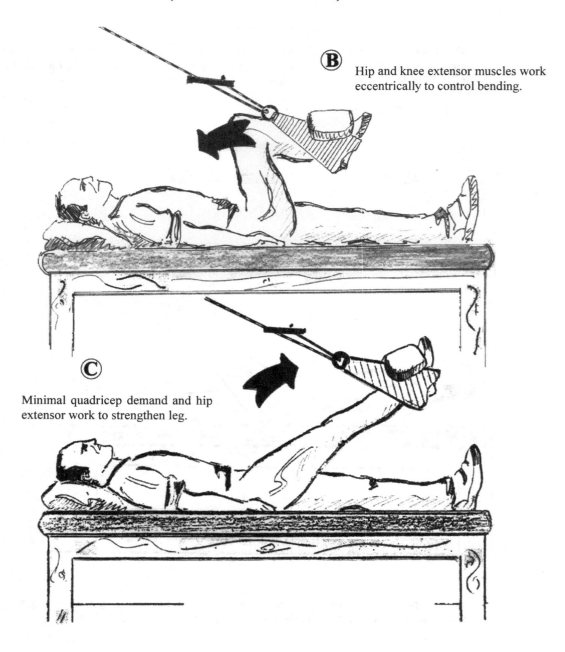

B Hip and knee extensor muscles work eccentrically to control bending.

C Minimal quadricep demand and hip extensor work to strengthen leg.

**Sling
Suspension
Therapy**

SUPINE LYING ASSISTED HIP FLEXION
(UTILIZING A PULLEY)

A   Illustrates the starting position
B   Illustrates the motion
C   Illustrates the return to the starting position

Pulling on the thigh sling (through the handle) initiates hip and knee flexion. This is a subtle movement. The overhead suspension point is above the head for the foot sling, and on the back suspension cage for the thigh (as illustrated)

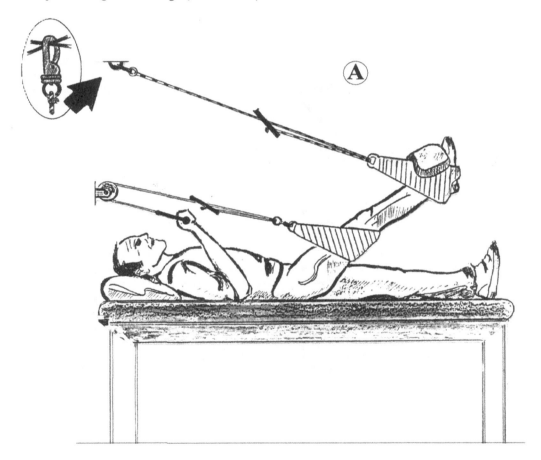

ASSISTED HIP FLEXION (UTILIZING A PULLEY)
(SUPINE LYING)

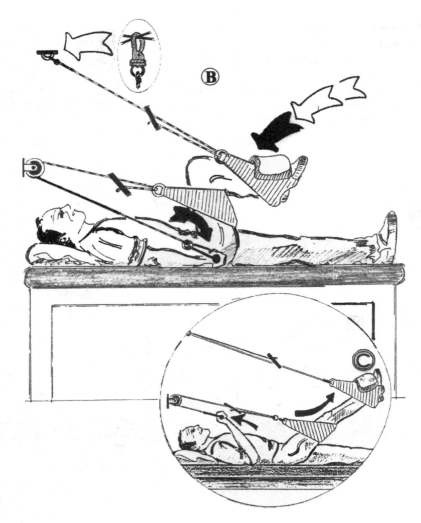

Quads work eccentrically lengthening under tension and acting like a slow brake to produce a smooth movement.

If the patient wishes to initiate knee flexion, this subtle technique will suffice. This is achieved by adding a simple cord and pulley (See illustration A).

**Sling
Suspension
Therapy**

SELF-ASSISTED, ACTIVE TENSION (SITTING)

The wood slat situated on the pulley cord provides the means of lengthening or shortening the cord. For this technique, there should be unobstructed clearance for the feet to move under the seat. When one leg begins to straighten it bends/flexes the opposite one. The technique illustrated should be executed smoothly with the goal of encouraging more knee flexion. Further knee flexion is encouraged by holding the knee flexed for 20-30 seconds. The thigh muscles primarily provide the power for this movement.

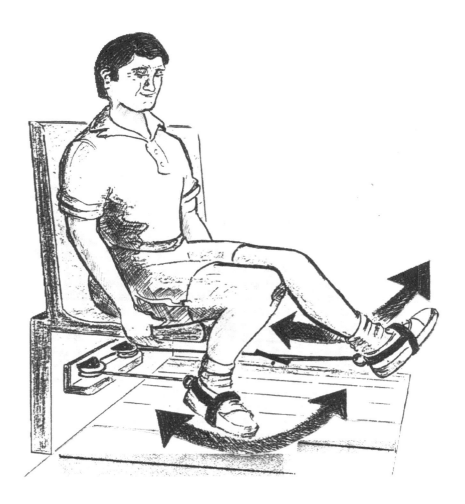

SELF-ASSISTED, ACTIVE TENSION (PRONE LYING)

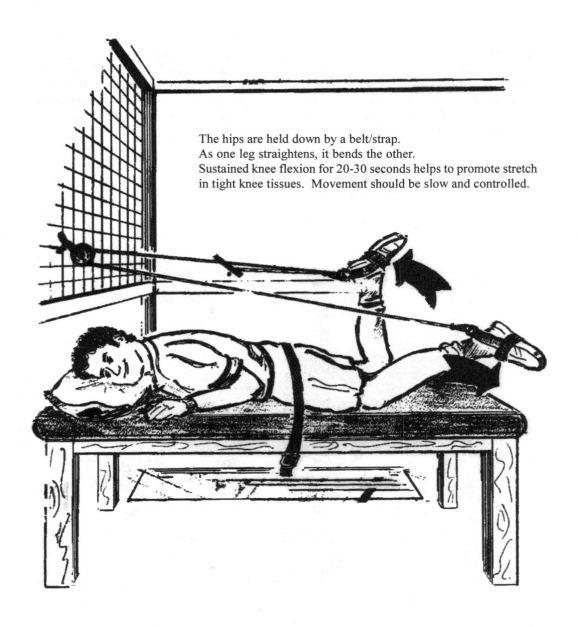

The hips are held down by a belt/strap.
As one leg straightens, it bends the other.
Sustained knee flexion for 20-30 seconds helps to promote stretch
in tight knee tissues. Movement should be slow and controlled.

PASSIVE, WEIGHT ASSISTED KNEE FLEXION PROLONGED STRETCH (SIDE LYING)

(A) Starting Position

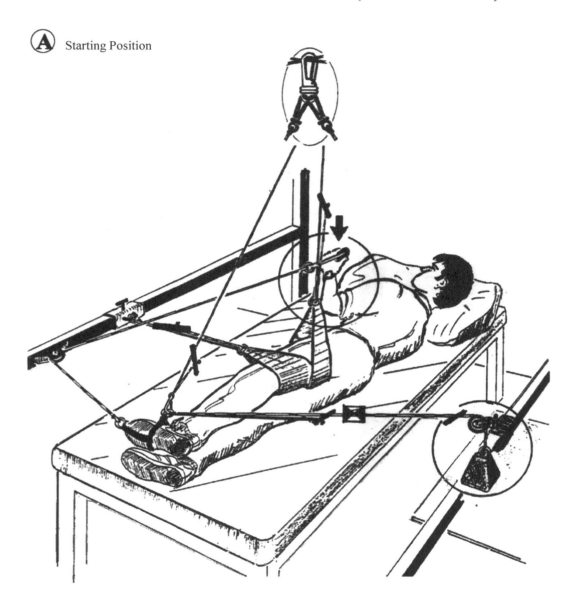

The common overhead suspension point is directly above the hip joint. The left hand/arm is holding the weight freeing up the left leg. The left thigh sling acts as a restraint to thigh movement.

Sling Suspension Therapy

PASSIVE, WEIGHT ASSISTED KNEE FLEXION PROLONGED STRETCH (SIDE LYING)

When the left elbow straightens, the pulley weight is transferred to the left foot facilitating weight assisted knee flexion. Tolerance to prolonged stretching of the thigh muscle (20 to 60 seconds) is determined by tissue discomfort and degree of quadriceps inter/intra muscle scarring.

(B) Weight is flexing the knee

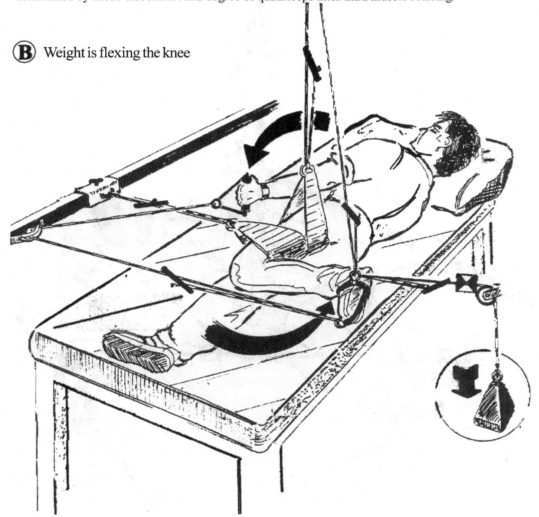

Although this technique presents some rigging challenges, practice runs will make one more familiar with the rigging and after slinging up a dozen people, the technique illustrated above will not seem so daunting to practice.

WEIGHT AND PULLEY RESISTED (SUPINE LYING)

This technique is an enjoyable way of strengthening the hamstring muscles. A tendency for the other leg to raise during strong hamstring work can be cured by strapping it down. In several suspension techniques, the therapist working with the patient can enhance the technique.

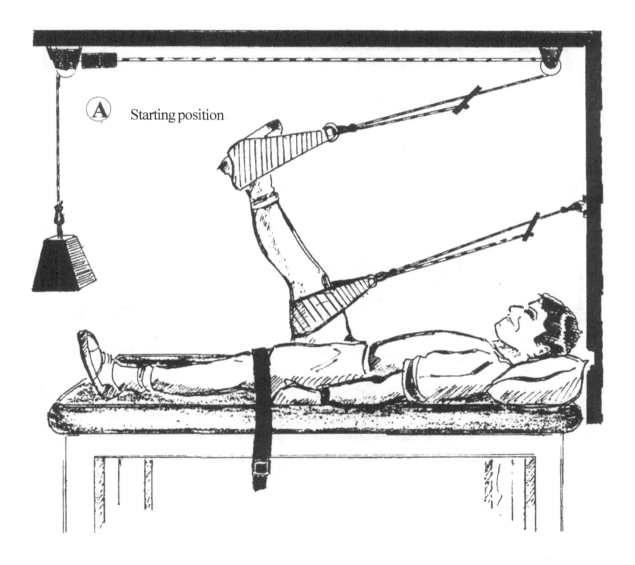

Ⓐ Starting position

WEIGHT AND PULLEY RESISTED (SUPINE LYING)

For most pulley work, the light plastic pulley is used . When dead weight is used(known as weight and pulley exercise) a heavier steel pulley is required.

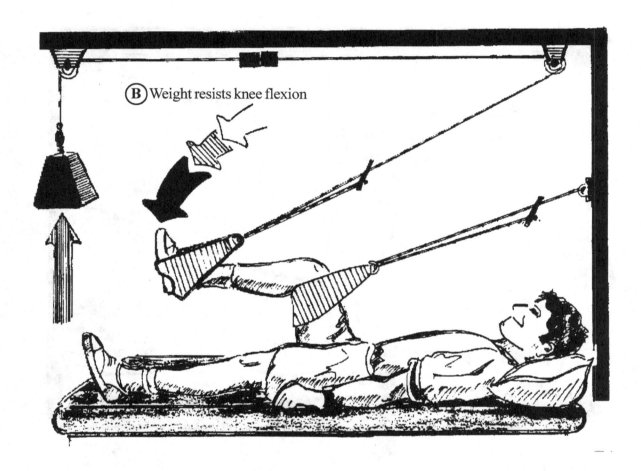

Ⓑ Weight resists knee flexion

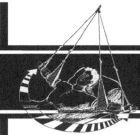

Foot & Ankle Series

Sustained weight assisted achilles/ankle joint stretch.

Sustained weight assisted foot-ankle plantar flexion (unilateral-bilateral)

**Sling
Suspension
Therapy**

SUSTAINED WEIGHT ASSISTED ACHILLES/ANKLE JOINT STRETCH

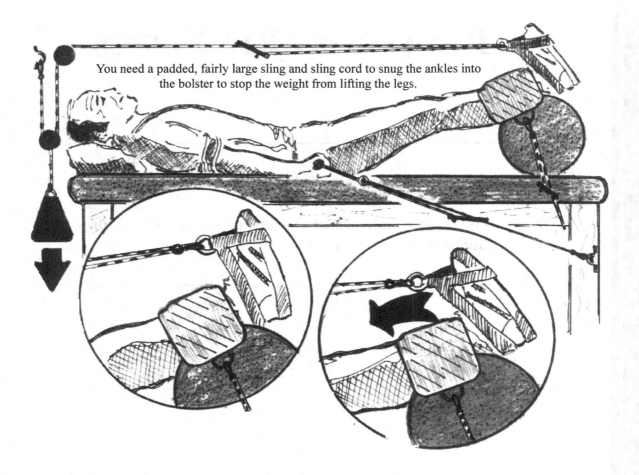

You need a padded, fairly large sling and sling cord to snug the ankles into the bolster to stop the weight from lifting the legs.

Primarily Weight Assisted Dorsi-Flexion Followed by Weight Resisted Plantar Flexion

a) Starting Position: Lying supine, both achilles tendons resting upon a bolster.
b) Equipment: Two foot/ankle sling straps
                   Two sets of pulleys and weights (twelve 10lb. weights)
                   One large spherical bolster or wedge, seat belt, one sling cord, one padded sling.

Sequence of Movement(s)

1. Activate calf muscles by plantar flexing feet. (push soles into foot slings)
2. Deactivate by allowing weight to assist in dorsi-flexion, resulting in Achilles tendon stretch.

Sling Suspension Therapy

SUSTAINED WEIGHT UNI/BILATERAL ANKLE/FOOT PLANTAR FLEXION

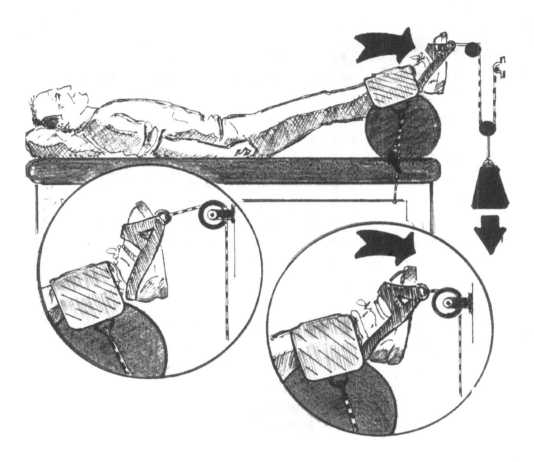

a) Starting Position: Supine Lying
b) Equipment: Two foot/ankle sling straps
                        Two sets of pulleys and weights (8 five pound.weights)
c) One large bolster, one sling cord, one padded sling.

Sequence of Movement(s)

1. Activate shin muscles by dorsi-flexing feet. (pulling forefeet towards shins)
2. Deactivate by allowing weight to pull feet back into plantar-flexion.

AMPUTEE THERAPY

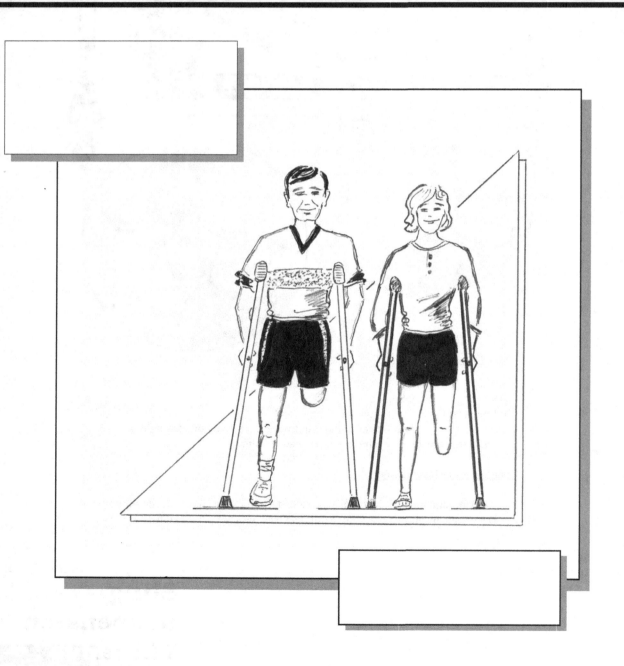

Contents

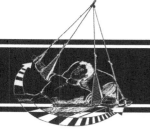

Amputee Therapy

Weight & Pulley Exercises

Several illustrated strengthening exercises specific to the below knee (BK) and above knee (AK). Amputee using sling suspension equipment.

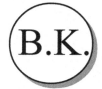

BELOW KNEE (B.K.)
Hip Abduction
Knee Extension
Knee Extension

ABOVE KNEE (A.K.)
Hip Adduction
Hip Extension
Hip Extension

Below Knee Amputee
Hip Abduction with Weight Resistance
Supine Posture

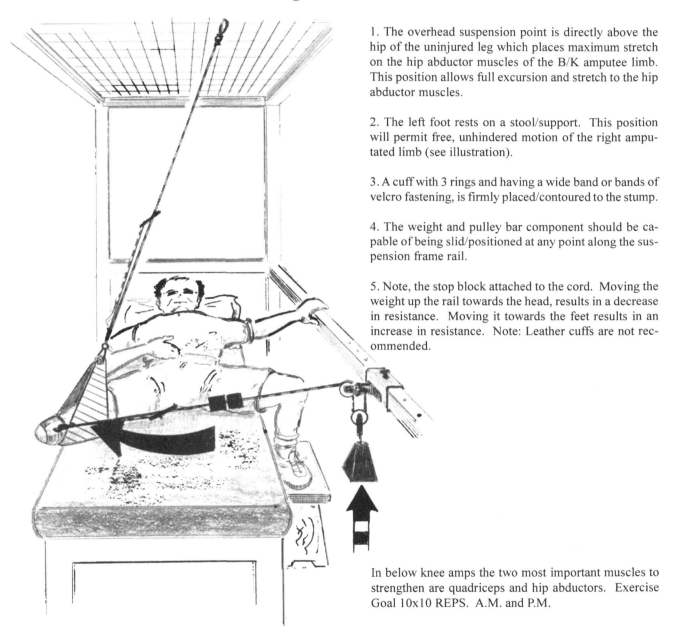

1. The overhead suspension point is directly above the hip of the uninjured leg which places maximum stretch on the hip abductor muscles of the B/K amputee limb. This position allows full excursion and stretch to the hip abductor muscles.

2. The left foot rests on a stool/support. This position will permit free, unhindered motion of the right amputated limb (see illustration).

3. A cuff with 3 rings and having a wide band or bands of velcro fastening, is firmly placed/contoured to the stump.

4. The weight and pulley bar component should be capable of being slid/positioned at any point along the suspension frame rail.

5. Note, the stop block attached to the cord. Moving the weight up the rail towards the head, results in a decrease in resistance. Moving it towards the feet results in an increase in resistance. Note: Leather cuffs are not recommended.

In below knee amps the two most important muscles to strengthen are quadriceps and hip abductors. Exercise Goal 10x10 REPS. A.M. and P.M.

Below Knee Amputee
Unilateral knee extension with weight resistance
Prone lying posture

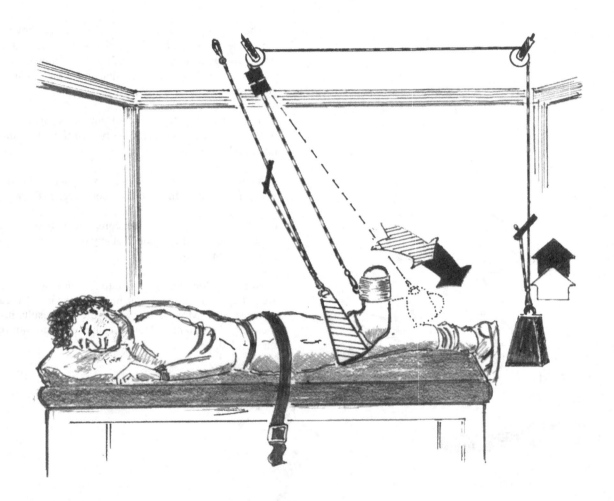

Notice the sling supporting the thigh and the belt securing the hips. Straightening of the leg results in strong contraction of the quadriceps muscle including the rectus femoris. Hip flexors to some degree work as fixator muscles. The stop block as it engages the pulley, carries the weight therby permitting the leg to relax. The sling that is slung below the left thigh holds the left thigh in full but comfortable hyperextension.

Below Knee Amputee
Unilateral knee extension with weight resistance
Inclined sitting posture

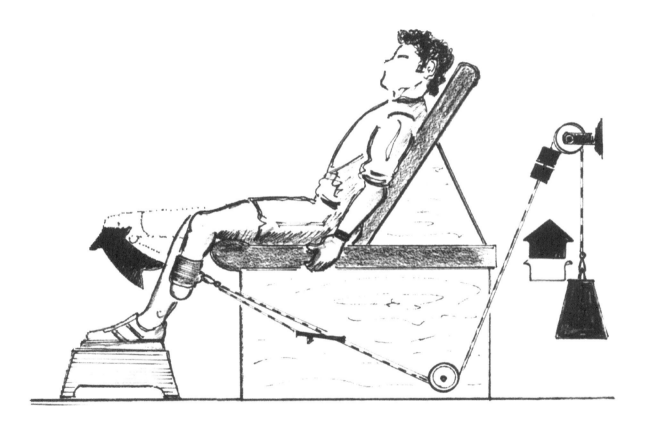

Note: When pulley and weight systems are used for strengthening muscles by Upper and Lower limb amputees, they should at all times, have the stump(s) bandaged and covered with either a cast sock, 1 ply or stockinette (sewn at one end to form a toe).

Starting Position: Sitting upon a special chair with an adjustable back support. The pulley and weight system should be clear of obstructions. The weight resistance exercise illustrated above strengthens the Quadriceps muscle using concentric then eccentric muscle work. To initiate knee extension, the amputee dorsi flexes the missing foot and follows this by straightening/extending the knee. The stump is held straight for 6 seconds then lowered.

Number of repetitions: At first 10 times, progress to 10 x 10 A.M. and P.M. A snug-fitting, adjustable cuff (That does not slip/ slide up and down the stump) is essential.

Above Knee Amputee
Unilateral hip adduction with weight resistance
Side lying posture

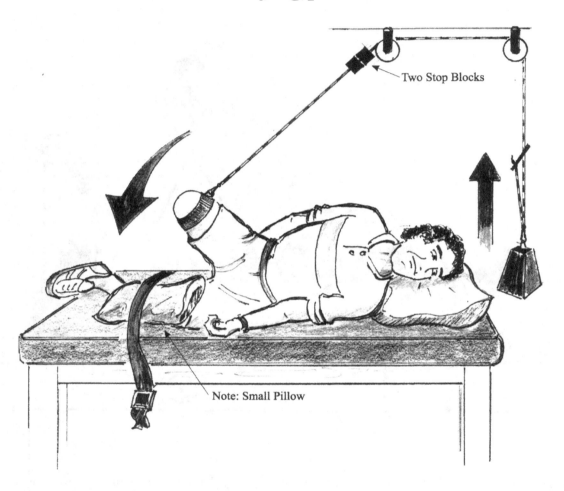

Two Stop Blocks

Note: Small Pillow

Hip adductor muscles arise off the pelvic rami inserting into the medial length of the femur. The shorter the stump the greater the loss of adductor muscle potential consequently the untouched gluteus medius and minimus dominate and tend to pull the stump into abduction. Likewise, loss of much of the hamstrings (powerful knee flexor but also a hip extensor) is no match for the psoas and iliacus (Hip Flexors) which pull the stump into flexion. Again, the external rotators of the hip dominate the weak internal rotators and the stump can end in abduction, flexion and external rotation. If allowed to stay in this position, contracture develop, thus in A/K amps, hyper strengthen the hip extensors, adductors and internal rotators.

Above Knee Amputee
Unilateral hip hyperextension with weight resistance
Supine posture

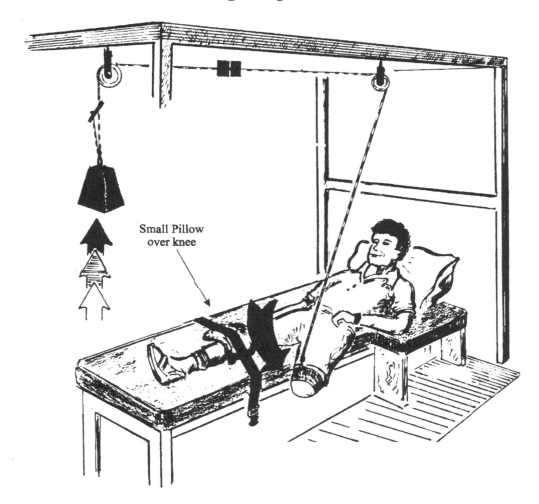

Small Pillow over knee

The overhead suspension point is approximately above the head, moving it towards the feet subtly increases the resistance. Note the pillow over the knee with the restraining strap over the pillow. The Gluteus Maximus muscle works to bring the stump into hyper-extension. To allow the stump to move comfortably through the whole range, the buttock must be clear of the plinth. This is important otherwise the hip will only reach extension. The hamstrings play some role in hyperextension of the stump. The shorter the stump, the less resistance. The hamstring contributes to the movement.

Above Knee Amputee
Unilateral hip hyperextension with weight resistance
Supine posture

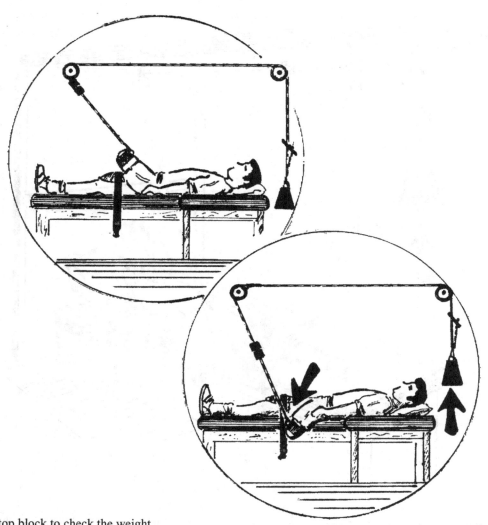

• Note the stop block to check the weight

• Excellent illustration of hip Hyperextension

• The stump cuff must not slip up or down the stump

INTRODUCTION

Progressive Physical Treatment

The content of this paper describes some physical treatment(s) available to the amputee (not discounting other aspects of their treatment during their period of rehabilitation.) The program is flexible and can be augmented or diminished. Many of the exercises have been illustrated which include Sling Suspension Therapy, Weight and Pulley and other activities listed herein. They allow the Physiotherapists to compile programs suitable for and tailored to each Amputees stage of recovery. The Rehabiliation system/program described in this text has consistantly produced outstanding, functional results in liason with the Amputee Team. This article may be used as a guide and source reference for those involved in the provision of physical treatment to Amputees. Special efforts are often called for both from the Physiotherapist and the amputee.

Additional information covering Amputations/ Amputees may be found in the Medical section of Physical Medicine Departments, Sports Medicine Departments, Hospital Rehabilitation Departments and the Medical Section of Hospitals and Public Libraries. A few books are listed in the Bibliography.

Brief Classification of Levels of Amputation
Upper and Lower Extremities

Upper Limb

Wrist disarticulation
Distal third trans radial (TR)
Middle third trans radial
Proximal third trans radial
Elbow diarticulation
Distal third trans humeral (TH)
Middle third trans humeral
Proximal third trans humeral
Shoulder disarticulation
Interscapulo-thoracio (IST)

Lower Limb

Ankle disarticulation (commonly Syme)
Distal third trans tibial (TT)
Mid third trans tibial
Proximal third trans tibial
Knee disarticulation
Distal third trans femoral (TF)
Mid third trans femoral
Proximal third trans femoral
Hip disarticulation
Hemi pelvectomy
Hemi corporectomy

Injury or disease may involve the upper or lower extremity at one or several places along the limb length. The extent of the disease or the severity of the injury will (among other factors) determine the need for amputation. The surgical procedure(s) used during amputation have an importatnt bearing upon whether the stump can be fitted comfortably with an Artificial Limb. Bones with sharp edges, loose muscle tissue flaps, sensitive sub-cutaneous nerve endings, once fairly common, are now, fortunately, seldom encountered due to improved surgical techniques. A more universal understanding also prevails with regard to the importance of an uncompromised blood supply to the skin flaps. Circum-stances permitting the surgical procedures of Myodesis and Myoplasty improve the muscles' function as a vascular pump and transmitter of motor power through the Prosthesis. It allows the Prosthetist to fabricate a snug-fitting socket.

Post Amputation Care

Following amputation and bed rest, the stump musculature is oedematous, atrophied and requires progressive exercise therapy. Lengthy use of a wheelchair and Axilla and Elbow crutches can result in a poor posture and there is a need to correct it. The stresses and strains of learning to cope with a Prosthesis are often exhausting. General conditioning of the body is considered to be a basic requirement. The anti-gravity muscles are given special attention to encourage a balanced standing posture. Exercises stressing mobility, strength, dexterity and endurance including balance and postural training need to be practiced daily. All muscle groups in proximity to the amputation site should also receive specific attention on a daily basis. The general conditioning aspect of the program should become a way of life, continuing after discharge from the Rehab Facility. Adequate time should be set aside each day (Monday to Friday inclusive) for practicing bandaging & stump hygiene procedures until proficiency has been acquired.

Use of a snug-fitting stump cuff when performing weight and pulley exercises is very important. Sad though it is to say, one has yet to see a well designed, safe, non-slip stump cuff for upper and lower limb stumps. Leather cuffs slip up and down the stump and can be a cause for discomfort to the amputee. Softer cuffs that mould better to the stump with rings and Velcro attachments are a step in the right direction, but leave room for improvement. One would think that this humble item (so very necessary) would have been fabricated years ago, but it hasn't changed since the dawn of time. It needs to be resolved. A vacuum or lace-up stump cuff is worthy of consideration.

Aims of Treatment

1) General

a) To develop, in the amputee, a physical readiness and general fitness condition that will result in excellent use and function of the Prosthesis with reference to a successful return to suitable employment

b) To develop, in the amputee, an awareness of how best to maintain an adequate, physical condition following discharge.

2) Specifics

a) Strengthening, mobilizing, conditioning
b) The complete Gait Training progressions for lower limb amputees
c) Education and practice in stump hygiene and bandaging
d) Proficiency in functional activities encountered in activities of daily living.

3) Progressive Exercise

a) Strengthening exercises specific to the amputation limb
b) Maintaining or restoring joint ranges when some of it is lost
c) Progressive functional activity (see page 104 for activities listed under "Final Phase of Gait Training")
d) Multiple amputation sites
e) General conditioning focussed primarily on the uninjured parts of the body
f) Hydro-Therapy
g) Selected games, activities ie: Table-tennis, darts, light air ball games, dancing etc. (see page 104 for activities listed under Final Phase of Gait Training)

Extremity Amputation

5) Bandaging

In the absence of a supporting plaster cast following amputation or following it's removal, stump tissues are best supported by Elastic Crepe Bandaging. Bandaging is almost an Art in itself and it takes much practice to apply one correctly so that the distal stump tissues receive adequate yet balanced tension which must lessen as the bandage wraps move proximally. If the bandage is applied too tightly it must be taken off and reapplied correctly. Any central or proximal constriction of the stump tissues through faulty bandaging can cause a tourniquet effect upon the blood and lymph vessels resulting in venous congestion, a tendency to distal swelling of the stump, and impairment of normal physiological function at cell level. It is worth an extra few words here to say that several efforts have been made in different regions of the World to fit stumps with so called stump shrinkers (which is a type of elastic stocking). In our experience these are a poor substitute for a well-applied elastic tensor bandage, and can even be the cause of some inconsiderable delay in the stump shrinkage.

As a rule of thumb we use:

i) 6 inch wide, elastic crepe bandages 10' to 15' long for bandaging above knee amputation stumps.
4 inch wide, elastic crepe bandages 5' to 10' long for bandaging below knee amputation stumps.
iii.) 3 inch or 4 inch wide, elastic crepe bandages 10' to 15' long for bandaging upper limb amputees.

The length of a bandage and the width used may vary. Common sense must reign as some amputated stumps are massive in size whilst others are small, but in general it is wiser to have more bandage than less. Elastic crepe bandages are usually 5 feet long, so it is necessary to join two or three of these together, dependant upon the requirements. The patient is taught how to bandage his/her stump correctly and most become quite proficient at it after 3 weeks or so.

Lower Extremity Amputation(s)

Bandaging:

A universally accepted method of bandaging an A/K and B/K stump is illustrated overleaf. The ideal way (and probably the only way) to acquire the skill for stump bandaging is to have an amputee therapist with practical experience teach it. From hereon in it is practice, practice and further practice until one has become proficient. Theory has it's place but practice achieves the desired result and improves on skill. Variations from the illustrated method of bandaging shown here are resorted to occasionally, however the basic principle of greatest support to the tissues distally must still be adhered to. Tubular Stockinette or a cast sock slipped over an awkward shaped, slippery stump, prior to bandaging may help the crepe bandage to grip and stay in place in cases when this is necessary. Incorrect bandaging might result in a Bulbous Stump End or Rabbit Ears or both. Using the Spica Method of Stump Bandaging (see illustration) decreases the chance(s) of this occuring. In active amputees the stump bandage can loosen and require re-wrapping. No <u>one</u> technique of stump bandaging / wrapping will fit all situations, although the Spica Wrap comes close to fulfilling this objective.

Above Knee or Through Knee Stump Bandaging

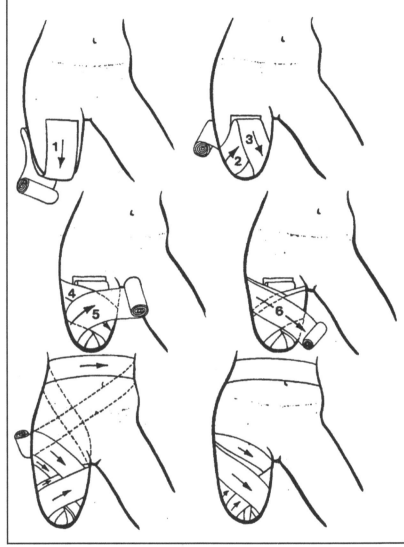

1. Place the end of the bandage anteriorly at the inguinal fold, the patient or assistant holding the two corners with his thumbs.

2. With the bandage at half stretch take it distally over the end of the stump and up the posterior aspect to the gluteal fold, the bandage is then held here by the patient's fingers. The next turn is taken again over the distal end of the stump slightly laterally and then returned anteriorly to the starting point, this turn again being held by the patient's thumbs.

3. Once more the third turn passes distally over the end of the stump, this time slightly medially. It is now passed proximally and laterally across the posterior aspect of the stump. It is held at this point and then brought diagonally downwards and medially across the anterior aspect (turn 4) and a turn is now taken firmly around the back of the stump at the distal end (turn 5).

4. Figure of eight turns are now continued around the stump working proximally until the whole of the stump has been covered and the turns taken well up into the groin.

5. A fixing turn is made by taking the bandage from the posterior aspect of the stump up over the buttock and then forward around the waist. It is best to have the patient turn on to the other side for this. As the turn is brought around the patient's back, he is asked to extend the stump. The bandage is then brought down again to the anterior aspect of the stump.

6. The rest of the bandage is used on one or two more turns on the stump, and fixed by two safety pins high up posterolaterally on the pelvis.

Below Knee Stump Bandaging

1. Place the end of the bandage anteriorly just below the tip of the patella, the patient or the assistant holding the two corners with his thumbs. With the bandage at half stretch take it distally over the end of the stump and up over the posterior aspect of the popliteal space. The bandage is held here by the patient's fingers.

2. The next turn is taken again over the distal end of the stump slightly laterally and then returns anteriorly to the starting point, this turn also now being held by the patient's thumbs.

3. Once more the third turn passes distally over the end of the stump, this time slightly medially. It is now passed proximally and laterally across the posterior aspect of the stump. It is held at this point and then brought diagonally downwards and medially across the anterior aspect (turn 4) and the turn now taken firmly around the back of the stump at the distal end (turn 5).

4. Figure of eight turns are now continued around the stump working proximally until the whole stump has been covered.

5. It is important not to put too much tension on the bandage or too many turns over the tibia as pressure sores can easily occur.

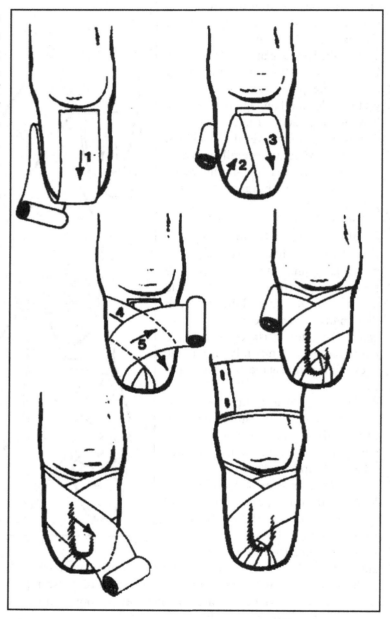

6. The bandage is finished by two or three turns above the knee. If the stump is short or the tibial shaft very superficial, the stump should be bandaged in extension and the knee joint included.

In what one might term conventional wrapping of the amputee stump (see illustration) it is not in contention that it is a good way to apply to a stump which can influence it's shape whilst maintaining physiological integrity. It is desirable that the first 2 or 3 wraps of the crepe/elastic bandage will support distal stump tissues by fashioning something akin to a sling prior to bringing about the next and classic figure of 8 herringbone wraps. To achieve this many amputees are taught to use their thumbs and fingers to hold the initial wraps. This is too often misapplied and negates the effect of bandaging. When stump conditions exist that prevent good conventional wrapping, the Dr. Kennard Spiker Wrap can be justified as it frees up the hands and permits better wrapping. The first 3 wraps act like a sling to the distal tissues and are the key and most important wraps when bandaging.

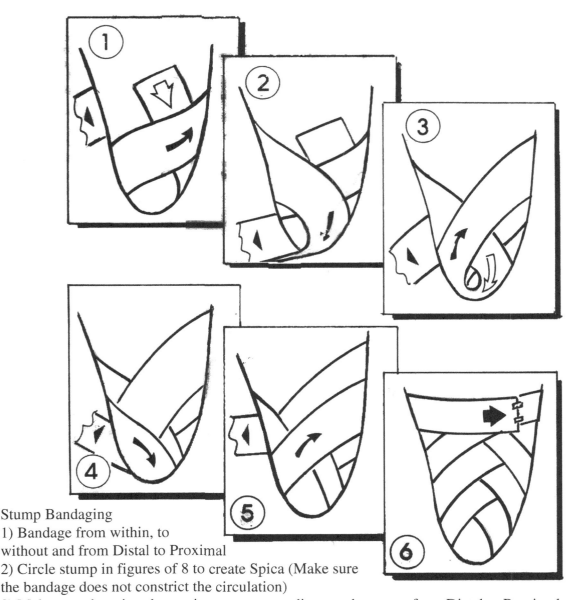

Stump Bandaging
1) Bandage from within, to without and from Distal to Proximal
2) Circle stump in figures of 8 to create Spica (Make sure the bandage does not constrict the circulation)
3) Make sure there is a decreasing pressure gradient up the stump from Distal to Proximal.
4) Finish with Fasteners making sure they are not positioned where they can cause areas of pressure.

Courtesy of Dr. A.B. Kennard M.B., B.S. (London)

Amputee Therapy

Extremity Amputation -cont.

6) Stump/Skin Care

The stump tissues should always be kept clean. Physohex or Hibitane will keep the skin healthy and aseptic. On hot days the stump should be washed and freshened up and exposed to the air for a spell. Stump socks should be changed daily, although in colder, northern climates, the stump sock may be worn for several days. The hotter the climate the more frequent the sock change, sometimes necessitating a midday change, once again common sense should prevail.

7. Upper Extremity Amputee

All upper limb amputees (especially above elbow) require good shoulder, shoulder girdle, neck and elbow (when applicable) joint mobility as well as strong muscle supports. The stump is inspected for healing, skin color and oedema and palpated for sensation or tender spots. The amputee is then instructed in stump bandaging and 2 or 3 weeks may pass before he/she achieves proficiency.

Shrinkage of any stump, be it upper or lower limb, usually occurs in two directions: 1) Circumferentially, and 2) Distal to Proximal. Stumps should remain bandaged when the Amputee is not wearing a Prosthesis including night-time, otherwise the stump tissues swell and may not fit comfortably into the socket in the morning. The bandage is removed intermittently to permit bathing etc. In general, until the Amputee is a good Prosthetic user or the stump has stabilized with regard to shrinkage, the stump should remain bandaged. In early stages of stump bandaging if there is too much stump pain at night-release the bandage for 20 minutes and then reapply. If pain recurs take the bandage off and leave it off until the morning. The amputee usually re-adapts to full use of the bandage by the 3rd or 4th night.

Upper Extremity Amputee

8. Specific Stump Exercises

The following exercises specific to Upper Extremity Amputation have been selected and are highly recommended for their excellent functional end results.

For the purpose of clarity these exercises can be classified into:
a) Early stage (for the beginning Upper Limb amputee) and consist of Free, Active, Exercise progressing to:
b) Final Stage that consists of Weight and Pulley resistance exercises.

9. Early Stage Specific, Free, Active Exercises (no equipment required)

a) Bilateral, active, elevation of shoulders Progress up to 3x10 repetitions
b) Bilateral, active, retraction of shoulders Progress up to 3x10 repetitions
c) Bilateral, active, protraction of shoulders Progress up to 3x10 repetitions
d) Bilateral, active, shoulder abduction of both arms to vertical Progress up to 3x10 repetitions
e) Bilateral, active, shoulder flexion of both arms to vertical Progress up to 3x10 repetitions
f) Actively attempt to place both hands behind and up the back 20 times
g) Actively attempt to place both hands behid the neck 20 times
h) Bilateral, active, elbow flexion and extension (Applies to below elbow amps)

10. Final Stage Specific Resistance Exercises Using Weight and Pulley Resistance (equipment required)

See pages 92 and 95 for illustrated, specific resistance, weight and pulley exercises

Some practice in the use of the Terminal Device on the Upper Limb Prosthesis is provided in the physiotherapy Department but the major part of Terminal Device instruction and practice is carried out by the Occupational Therapist including activities of Daily Living.

Some emphasis on visualizing phantom limb and it's normality can be included in the Amputees Program.

Amputee - Upper Limb - Weight and Pulley Exercise

A1   Resisted Bilateral Shoulder Retraction
A2   Resisted Bilateral Shoulder Protraction
A3   Resisted Bilateral Shoulder Elevation
A4   Resisted Unilateral Elbow Flexion
A5   Resisted Unilateral Elbow Extension
A6   Resisted Unilateral Arm and Shoulder Extension
A7   Resisted Unilateral Arm and Shoulder Flexion
A8   Resisted Unilateral Arm Adduction Whilst at 90° Flexion / Protraction
A9   Resisted Unilateral Arm Abduction Whilst at 90° Flexion / Retraction

Amputee Therapy

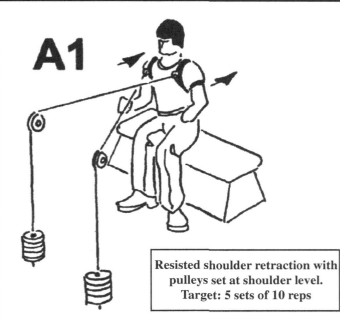

A1

Resisted shoulder retraction with pulleys set at shoulder level.
Target: 5 sets of 10 reps

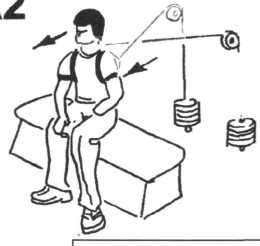

A2

Resisted shoulder protraction
Target: 5 sets of 10 reps

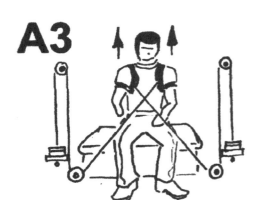

A3

Resisted shoulder girdle elevation
Target: 5 sets of 10 reps

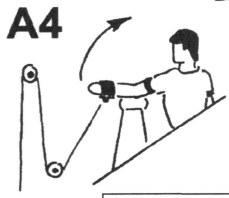

A4

Resisted elbow flexion
with arm support
Target: 5 sets of 10 reps

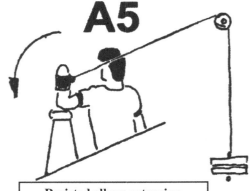

A5

Resisted elbow extension
with arm support
Target: 5 sets of 10 reps

Amputee Therapy

Specific Resisted Exercises for the Upper Limb Amputee

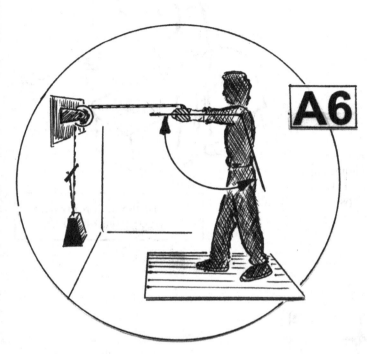

A6- Resisted Arm/Shldr Extension

The wall pulley is at shoulder height. Face pulley-one leg ahead opposite arm is straight and held in 90° of shoulder flexion. The arm cuff must fit securely and comfortably and support the stump tissues. The stump tissues demand excellence in bandaging. Exercise: Pull the arm down and a little behind torso. (See A6 Illus.) Repetitions: Initially 10 times progressing to 5 sets of 10 reps.

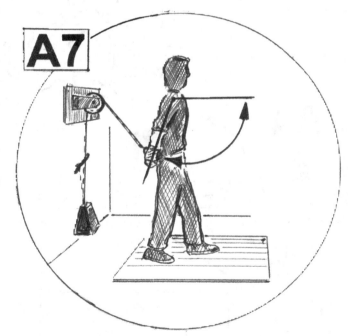

A7- Resisted Arm/Shldr Flexion

The wall pulley is at shoulder height. Present back to pulley (see illus.) If amputation is to right arm place left foot forward and vice versa. Clip the pulley cord to the arm cuff and adjust cord length (if required) so that the straight arm lies just beyond the hip in hyperextension. Exercise: Pull straight arm forwards achieving 90° of shoulder flexion. Repetitions: Initially 10 reps progressing to 5 sets of 10 reps.

Specific Resisted Exercises for the Upper Limb Amputee

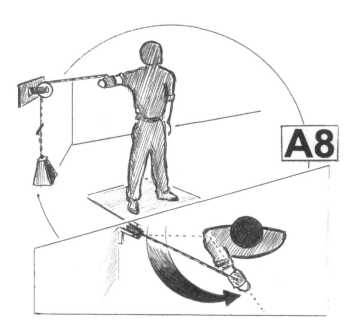

Resisted Adduction/Protraction

Standing side-on to wall pulley, pulley wheel level with shoulder, injured arm at 90° abduction and clipped to the amputee exercise cuff. Exercise: Keeping arm at shoulder level and straight adduct/Protract it across the chest (see illustration). Repetitions: At first 10 times progressing to 5 sets of 10.

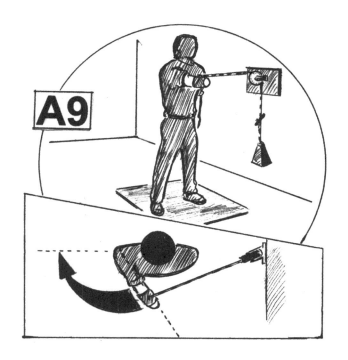

Resistance to shoulder retractor muscles

The arm moves out sideways starting at 90° flexion & ending in 90° adduction standing - side on to wall pulley facing the complete opposite direction to A8 above. Pulley wheel level with shoulder.(see A9 illustration) Repetitions: At firt 10 times progressing to 5 sets of 10.

Upper Limb
Requirements for Discharge Status

a)   Patient can demonstrate good, functional use and control of the prosthesis and terminal device.

b)   Patient demonstrates good range of movement and power in joints and muscles of the shoulder and elbow (Below elbow amp)

c)   Comfortable Prosthetic Socket Fit

d)   Stump shrinkage complete

e)   Is proficient in applying and removing the prosthesis especially where a harness is involved.

f)   There is no oedema, pain or skin discoloration after wearing/using the prosthesis all day.

g)   Is proficient at pulling the stump fully into suction socket using a pull sock.

There should be no oedematous tissues, induration, discoloration, lymphatic or vascular impairment after participating in any of the "CRITERIA FOR DISCHARGE" activities listed above.

**Amputee - Lower Limb - Free, Active and Weight
and Pulley Exercises**

A1   Supine - Below Knee Amp - Straighten Knee Quadricep Work
A2   Supine - Above Knee Amp - Stump Hyperextension (hip)
A3   Side Lying - B/K or A/K Amp Hip/Stump Abduction
A4   Prone Lying Lift Head and Trunk Hip and Back muscle work
A5   Standing between adjustable parallel bars Pulley and weight Adductor work
A6   Standing between adjustable parallel bars Pulley and Weight Hip hyperextension work
A7   Standing between adjustable parallel bars Pulley and weight Pull stump sideways
A8   Using Axilla crutches, standing Weight and Pulley Keep knee straight Pull Forwards
A9   Lying Supine Use shiny board Good foot on stool Abductor and Adductor leg
A10   Sitting Weight and Pulley Straighten knee Concentric muscle work for thigh

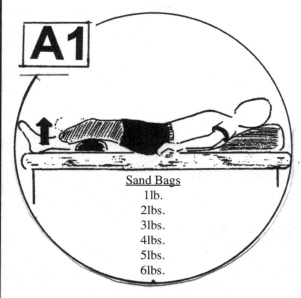

Below Knee Amputation

Some specific stump exercises to strengthen knee extensors and hip abductors in the lying, sitting and standing position. Supine Lying - Strengthening of Quadriceps (knee extensors) acting upon stump. Starting position a) Small pad beneath knee (see diagram). Movement(s) Concentric Muscle Work b) Dorsi-flex amputated foot, then raise distal end of stump until knee is staight, hold this position for 6 seconds, then return to starting position. (see diagram) If painful chondromalcia is present, remove pad and modify the exercise by performing a straight leg raise. (Isometric quads work).

Number of times c) at first 10 times. Goal d) ten sets of 10 repetitions. Note: Greater demand upon the latent power inherent in the quadriceps muscle may be activated by the judicious use of sand-bags or therapist resistance.

Sand Bags
1lb.
2lbs.
3lbs.
4lbs.
5lbs.
6lbs.

Above Knee Amputation

Some specific stump exercises to strengthen hip extensors and hip abductors in the lying, sitting and standing position. Supine Lying - Strengthening of Gluteus Maximus and hamstrings (hip extensors) acting upon stump. Starting position a) Lying supine upon a firm, comfortable, support normal leg bent at knee to allow the foot to rest comfortably upon the supporting surface the A/K stump rests in a natural position. Movement(s) Concentric Muscle Work for Hip Extensors b) raise normal knee towards the chest, grasping it in both hands (knee joint is fully flexed) then actively extend the A/K stump attempting to achieve 15° hyperextension at the hip joint, hold, and then return to the starting position to permit muscle relaxation. Number of times c) at first 10 times. Goal d) ten sets of 10 repetitions.

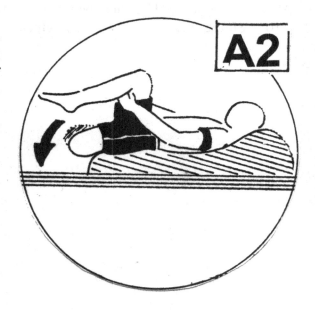

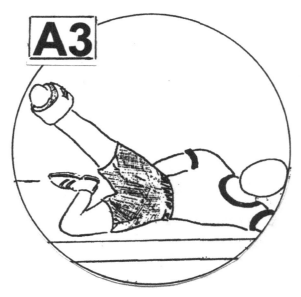

Hip Abductor

Lying on the side upon a plinth
Strengthening of hip abductors. Starting Position a) Lying on side upon plinth; lower knee and hip well flexed to provide lateral body stability uppermost leg is straight and in line with the trunk. Movement(s) Concentric Muscle Work for Abductors b) keeping the leg straight, raise it sideways and upwards to a maximum, yet not uncomfortable height, followed by leg lowering to the starting position. Number of times c) at first 10 times. Goal d) ten sets of 10 repetitions Note: Progress in strength by adding a light sand bag striving for the optimum weight of 15 lbs.

Spine & Hip Extensors

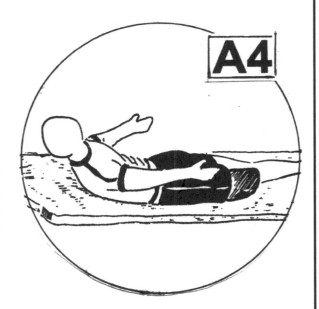

Prone Lying
Strengthening of gluteus maximus and hamstrings (indirect) Starting position a) Lying prone (face down) upon a mat, face turned to one side, shoulders relaxed, arms internally rotated and palm of hands facing the ceiling. Movement(s) Inner range muscle work (concentric and static) for spinal and hip extensors b) raise head and trunk; simultaneously externally rotating the shoulders to turn the palm of the hands outwards, hold for 2 seconds then return to starting position. Number of times c) at first 10 times. Goal d) three sets of 10 repetitions

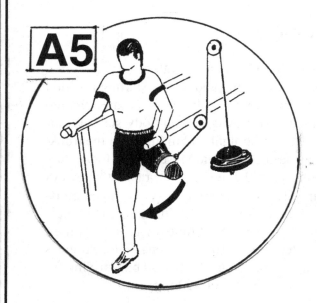

Standing

Strengthening of hip adductors
Starting Position-a)Standing upright upon normal leg facing towards (and both hands holding onto) chair back the A/K stump is held in full abduction through tension on the weighted pulley cord. Movement(s) Concentric muscle work for hip adductors b) Pull A/K stump downwards and medially to press against normal leg. Number of times-c) at first 10 times. Goal d) Ten sets of 10 repetitions.

Standing

Strengthening of hip extensors
Starting Position a)Standing upright between two chairs, hands holding chairs to stabilize trunk stump is flexed to approx. 90°. Movement(s) concentric muscle work b) Attempt to pull A/K stump back into hyperextension. Number of times c) At first 10 times. Goal d) Ten sets of 10 repetitions.
Note: Sometimes this exercise can be carried out in the sitting position. The therapist should be alert to any lower back problems.

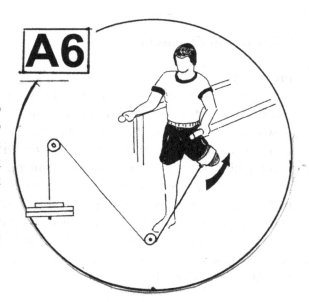

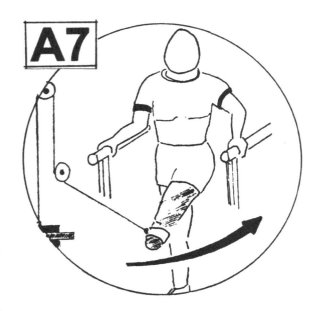

Standing

Strengthening of hip abductors
Starting position. a) Standing upright upon norml leg hands holding onto a chair back to stabilize trunk stump lies in front of normal leg and medially adducted   Movement(s) Concentric muscle work for Gluteus Medius, Minimus and Tensor Fascia Lata   b) Maintaining a comfortable, upright posture, the stump is moved laterally. The B/K stump passes in front of the normal leg during its lateral excursion. Number of times c) At first 10 times Goal d) Ten sets of 10 repetitions.

Standing

Strenghtening of quadriceps (knee extensors) acting upon stump isometric muscle work. Starting Position a) "USING AXILLA CRUTCHES" (adjusted to the correct length) for stabilizing the body during the performance of the exercise, have patient stand upright upon the sound leg facing away from the apparatus. Movement(s) Isometric Muscle Work for Quadriceps Concentric Muscle Work for Hip Flexors b) Whilst maintaining an upright posture with the aid of Axilla Crutches, the patient performs the following successive sequences of movements: i) Dorsi-flexion of the amputated foot ii) Static contraction of the quadriceps muscle acting upon the stump (to prevent knee flexion) iii) Downward / forward / upward motion of the amputated lower limb followed by immediate return to the starting position. Note: The motion should be performed smoothly. The knee should not be allowed to bend during any part of the movement, as the exercise is primarily to strengthen the knee extensor. Lifting the amputated limb too high IN FRONT of the body should be DISCOURAGED the leg should NOT be stopped at the limit of its forward swing but allowed to return IMMEDIATELY.

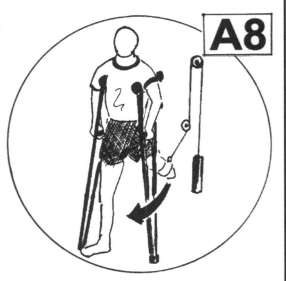

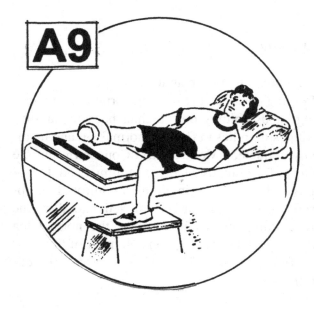

Abductors/Adductors

Supine on Plinth
Strengthening of hip abductors (and adductors). Starting Position: a) Lying supine upon plinth normal leg abducted sufficiently enough to allow the knee to bend and permit the foot to rest upon a stool the stump (with bandage or stump sock on) rests upon the surface of a wide rectangular "SHINY SURFACED" board. Movement(s): Concentric muscle work for Abductors and Adductor. b) Slide the stump from side to side across the shiny-surfaced board. Stump should swing through as wide an arc as possible promoting maximum abduction (and adduction) of the hip. Number of times: c) At first 20 consecutive times without weight (add 5 lb. sand bags progressing to a maximum of 35 lbs.). Goal: d) Ten sets of 20 repetitions.

Knee Extensors

Sitting
Strengthening of quadriceps (knee extensors) acting upon stump, using a weight and pulley resistance. To ensure care of stump tissues and to facilitate this form of quads resistance using a good fitting cuff is necessary. Starting Position: a) Sitting upon a stout chair legs relaxed (see diagram). Movement(s) Concentric muscle work: b) Dorsi-flex amputated foot, then pull stump forward/upward until the knee is straight, hold this position for 6 seconds, then return to starting position. (see diagram). Contra-indication painful chondromalcia. Number of times: c)At first 10 times. Goal: d) Ten sets of 10 repetitions

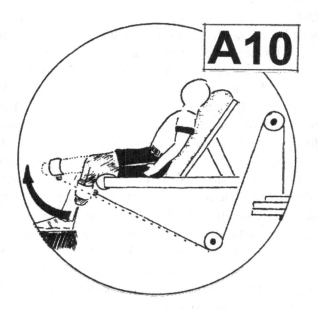

AMPUTEE GAIT TRAINING GUIDE

<u>Below Knee Amputation (Gait Training Guide)</u>

<u>Item 1</u>: Instruct patient in stump and stump sock hygiene

<u>Item 2</u>: Instruct patient in stump bandaging use 4" wide elastic crepe bandage. 10 feet long is usually sufficient.

<u>Item 3</u>: Instruct patient in stump exercises SPECIFIC TO: Knee extensors (quadriceps) and abductors (gluteus medius etc.) in:
   a) lying
   b) sitting
   c) standing

<u>Item 4</u>: Instruct patient in general fitness program NON-SPECIFIC

<u>Item 5</u>: EARLY PHASE OF GAIT TRAINIG (using parallel walking bars)
   a) Check patient's stump, stump socket and stump socks
   b) Check patient's leg length whilst wearing the B/K prosthesis in supine lying and standing
   c) Check patient's leg length when the foot of the normal leg is standing upon a raised block.
   d) Check patient's toe alignment.
   e) Check patient's crutches for correct length.
   f) Instruct patient in parallel walking bars in balanced standing practice shifting weight from one leg to the other. Swaying.
   g) Instruct patient in parallel walking bars, one foot forward hands holding bars practice shifting body weight from one leg to the other.
   h) Instruct patient in parallel walking bars, walking one pace check posture and coordination of body segments.
   i) Instruct patient in parallel walking bars, practice walking in parallel bars using both hands
   j) Instruct patient in parallel walking bars, practice walking in parallel bars using one or either hand.
   k) Instruct patient in parallel walking bars, practice walking for short spells using lighter hand support.
   l) Instruct patient in parallel walking bars, devote longer periods of time to continuous walking.

<u>NOTE:</u> Check stump tissues for pressure points regularly.

The above <u>EARLY PHASE of GAIT TRAINING</u> is very important and may necessitate spending up to two weeks or longer to learn how to ambulate confidently with balanced gait and upright posture using a temporary B/K prosthesis before progressing out of the parallel walking bars to the <u>intermediate phase of gait training.</u>

<u>Item 6</u>: <u>Intermediate phase of Gait Training</u> (parallel walking bars discontinued)
   a) Using crutches teach patient normal walking.
   b) Using crutches teach patient and have him practice sitting down on to a chair and vice versa.
   c) Using crutches teach patient and have him practice getting down onto the floor and vice versa.
   d) Using crutches teach patient and have him practice ascending and descending stairs/steps.

e) Using crutches teach patient and have him practice ascending and descending slopes and ramps of varying degrees.

f) Using crutches teach patient and have him practice 90 degree pivot turns to left and right (subject to stump tissues permitting)

g) Using crutches teach patient and have him practice side stepping.

h) Using crutches devote longer periods of time to continuous walking.

NOTE: Check stump tissue for pressure points regularly.

Item 7: Gait training using two canes (Use of crutches discontinued)

a) Using two canes repeat all of the activities in 6 above

b) Practice different combinations of walking with canes and walking with one cane.

c) Introduce some activities requiring more balance, concentration and coordination control, when patient's gait is confident and stump free of pressure points such as:

    i)   Stepping up or over simulated street curbs.

    ii) Balance along straight lines or circles.

    iii) Dribbling a ball using the hand or a hockey stick.

    iv) Walks to local shops and parks.

    v) Blindfold patient and ask him to walk in the direction he hears your voice coming from.

Item 8: Final phase of Gait Training (use of canes discontinued)

Introduce more activities, taking into account walking ability, stump condition, prosthetic fit, age and general fitness.

Note: Some of these activities are fairly advanced. Use discretion in selecting the activity.

a) Walking practising 180 degree pivot-type turns

b) Shuffleboard

c) Ascending and descending a long flight of stairs with unbroken rhythm

d) Ascending and descending slopes

e) Walking bouncing a ball first with one hand, then the other

f) Balancing along the rib of B.E. benches

g) Stepping over a string of obstacles

h) Table tennis

i) Hop/skip running

j) Skipping

k) Obstacle course

l) Dancing

m) Badminton

n) General fitness circuit

Note:

1. Check stump tissues for pressure points regularly.

2. Prior to discontinuance of crutches and canes, the amputee will have progressed from 4 point to 3 point to 2 point walking

3. The amputee in using walking aids should work with 2 Axilla Crutches or 2 forearm/elbow crutches or 2 canes and finally no canes. One walking aid should never be used as it lends itself to a faulty posture and a disrythmic gait. It's either 2 walking aids or none at all, rarely an exception to this rule.

Amputee Therapy

Above Knee Amputation (Gait Training Guide)

The progressive method suggested for training below knee amputees in the re-education of walking (see Sheet No. 103 and 104) and use of their prosthesis may also be applied to above knee amputees with the following exceptions/additions.

1. Instruct patient in stump exercises SPECIFIC TO: hip extensors (gluteus maximums etc.) and hip adductors in:
   a) lying
   b) sitting
   c) standing

2. Therapist will probably need to bandage the A/K stump until the patient becomes skilled enough to bandage his own. Use 6" wide elastic crepe bandages, 15 feet plus or minus. Better to have too much bandage than too little.

3. If a suction (suspension) socket is worn as the definite prosthesis; the patient will need to be taught how to pull the stump tissues into the socket by using a pull sock (a length of stockinette serves well). Constant daily practice should eventually lead to the stump tissues being pulled fully into the suction socket and correctly seated. This is very important. Remove the socket valve and thread pull sock through valve hole.

4. a) With patient using crutches, teach him to practice sitting down onto a chair and vice versa.
   b) With patient using crutches, teach him to practice getting down on the floor and vice versa.

5. If the prosthesis possesses a knee-lock, teach the patient how to use it

6. Above knee amputees are not able to ascend stairs and steps one leg following the other. Teach amputee to ascend stairs and steps with the sound limb always leading. It is a rarity indeed for one to meet an A/K amputee able to ascend stairs or steps using alternate legs (at least at the present time).

7. Teach the patient how to take care of his prosthesis. If the definite prosthesis has hydraulic knee and ankle components, teach the amputee how to adjust the knee cadence and dorsi or plantar-flex the foot.

8. Note: In Sheet No. 103 & 104 "Below Knee Amputations" (see attached), under item 8 Final Phase of Gait Training (Use of canes discontinued), a list of activities is provided that requires a fairly high degree of skill, dexterity, balance, coordination and numerous postural changes whilst the body is in motion, which while obtainable goals for some below knee amputees is far more difficult for many above knee amputees, although a fair percentage of the activities listed in Item 8 are obtainable activities for above knee amputees, given time, practice and determination.

It is reiterated that a Progressive Method (Sheet No. 103 & 104 attatched; Items 1 to 8 included) suggested for training below knee amputees in the re-education of walking, is also applicable to the re-education of walking to above-knee amputees with the exceptions/additions as described above.

It is very important that when the amputee is in the standing position with the stump tissues fully seated in the socket, that the leg length is equal and the pelvis level, otherwise back problems may be precipitated if the prosthesis is short or too long.

The above "CRITERIA FOR DISCHARGE" cannot be met by all amputees. Bilateral and Multiple Amputation with possible multiple injury involvement, pose problems of balance and function that leave no other choice but the use of one or two canes or above elbow crutches to offset the otherwise high risk factor of falling and re-injury. A longer period of accommodation to socket wear and ambulation after physical rehabilitation has accomplished its purpose will alone determine less need to rely upon aids.

Lower Limb
Requirements for Discharge Status

a)   Amputee can demonstrate good, functional use and control of the prosthesis.

b)   Amputee can demonstrate maximum, potential range of movement and power in joints and muscles of lower limb.

c)   Comfortable Prosthetic / Socket Fit

d)   Stump shrinkage is complete.

e)   Is proficient in applying and removing the prosthesis.

f)   There is no oedema, pain or skin discoloration after wearing/using a lower limb prosthesis all day.

g)   Is well versed in the use of the pull-sock to achieve maximum entry of the stump into the socket.

h)   Has acquired confidence in adjusting the cadence and stride length by altering the resistance of the ankle and knee hydraulics mechanism.

Phys•Functional Evaluation of the AMPUTEE patient

NAME	
AGE	
OCCUPATION	
TYPE OF AMPUTATION	AIDS
GENERAL CONDITION (1-5)	

LOWER LIMB	BALANCE STATUS (1-5)			
	WALKING STATUS (1-5)			
	HIP	FLEXION		
		EXTENSION		
		ABDUCTION		
		ADDUCTION		
	KNEE	FLEXIONS 'STATIC'		
		EXTENSIONS		

UPPER LIMB	B. ELBOW	FLEXION		
		EXTENSION		
	A. ELBOW	PROTRACTION		
		RETRACTION		
		ELEVATION		
	SHOULDER	ABDUCTION		
		ADDUCTION		
		FLEXION		
		EXTENSION		

STUMP MEASURE-MENTS					

* GENERAL CONDITION *

SIT-UPS		STAIRS		
SQUATS		RAMPS		
PUSH-UPS		OBSTACLES		
CURLS		DISTANCE WALK		
BENCH PRESS		WALK W/ WEIGHT		
EXTENSIONS				

SPECIAL CONCERNS

REPORTING   ATTENDANCE

SUBJECTIVE FINDINGS

OBJECTIVE FINDINGS

ASSESMENT

PLAN

_____
_____
_____
_____
_____
_____
_____
_____
_____
_____
_____
_____
_____
_____
_____
_____
_____
_____
_____
_____

REVIEW RECOMMENDATION

THERAPIST_____
              DATE _____

Amputee Therapy

107

Conclusion

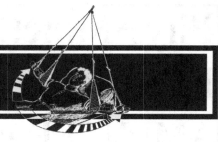

The Future-Passing the Knowledge On

Schools of learning that teach a body of knowledge, which might become a discipline exist to spread that body of knowledge worldwide and from generation to generation.

Wherever in the world that physiotherapy training facilities exist, be they at University hospitals or Colleges, it is hoped that faculty of such schools and the teachers of physiotherapy will find this Manual of Illustrated Sling and Cord Suspension Therapy Techniques useful reference work to draw upon. The contents of this book are entirely original work.

Sling Suspension Therapy can encompass a wide spectrum of techniques and developing it to it's greatest potential will require greater attention to engineering design. Better use of modern pulleys, plastics and metal matrixes might result in improved equipment. In addition, the fabric and design of slings (padded or otherwise) can be improved and require a more thoughtful approach than in the past.

Amputee Therapy

Index

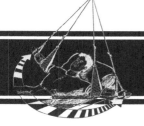

Bibliography

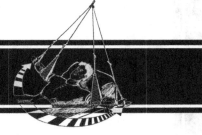

The Principals of Exercise Therapy, By Dena Gardiner, F.C.S.P. 3rd Edition, 1964, pub. G. Bell & Sons Ltd., London.

Tidy's Massage and Remedial Exercises, By J.O. Wale-11th edition,1968, pub. John Wright & Sons Ltd, Bristol.

Clinical Kiniesiology, By Signe Brunnstrom M.A.-3rd edition, reprinted May 1980, pub. F.A. Davis Company.

Physics Made Simple, By A. Howard & Wyndham Company, Reprinted May 1980, pub. Andrew H Allen & Co, London.

Amputees Guide-Below the Knee
Published in Co-operation with Prosthetic Research Study Seattle, Washington, operating under terms of Veterans Administration Contract No. V5261P-438
Foreword by Ernst M. Burgess M.D.
Principle Investigator Prosthestic Research Study
Medic Publishing Co P.O. Box 1636, Bellvue, Washington, USA
98009

The Management of Lower Extremity Amputations (TR10-6 August 1969)
Surgery
Immediate Postsurgical Prosthetic Fitting
Patient Care
       Ernst M. Burgess M.D., Principal Investigator
       Robert L Romano M.D., Associate Investigator
       Joseph H. Zettl, CP., Director
       Prosthetics Research Study
       Seattle, Washington, USA

This Publication was prepared for the prosthetic and sensory aids service
Veterans Administration under the terms of contract No. V5261P-438
Library of Congress Catalog card No.70-602818
For Sale by the Superintendant of Documents, U.S. Government
Printing Office-Washington, D.C. 20402 Price $1.50

Prosthetic and Sensory Aids Service
Department of medicine and Surgery
Veterans Administration, Washington DC

Pre-Prosthetic Care for Below Knee Amputees, 2nd Edition-Rehab. Institute of Chicago

Pre-Prosthetics Care for Above Knee Amputees, 2nd Edition-Rehab. Institute of Chicago

Rehabilitation of the Lower Limb Amputee - by W. Humm M.S.R.G.
Baillier, Tindal & Cassell Ltd. (7-8 Henrietta Street) W.C.2 England 2nd Edition 1968

Amputee Therapy

Footnote

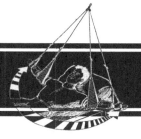

SPRINGS

You may have noticed that a resting spring has a loose piece of cord running through it's center. When a spring is stretched to the point where the slack in the cord is entirely taken up, the poundage resistance stamped upon the metal tab at one end of the spring has been reached. Springs can be used in Parallel or in Series (linked together like sausages).

Springs are available in 5 lb. increments ranging from 5lbs. to 50 lbs. and beyond. One of the negative aspects about Springs (to coin a phrase) is their penchant to unruliness, their springiness running wild.

A muscle whose fibres are fully stretched is said to be in a physiologically sound position to contract in but springs can upset this by offering maximum resistance when the muscle fibres are in their shortest position.

Example: Biceps, an elbow flexor. The constantly increasing resistance, as the spring(s) stretch can be quite challenging and unsettling, especially where repetitions are involved. We have used springs sparingly and with descretion in this manual. An uncontrolled snap-back from a stretched spring can sometimes exacerbate tissue that is on the mend.

Printed in the United States
by Baker & Taylor Publisher Services